The Shift.
Own Your Emotions;
Own Your Life.

BY
Gabrielle D. Lilly, MA

DEDICATION:

For Jacob, Justice, Harmony, Moses, Ben, Adam, Bo,
and all present and future
parents and children of parents.

Many thanks to all the people and other beings who
or that have conspired on my behalf.

Thank you to

This body.
This Universe.
All Potential Multiverses.
All things dark and sweet.
All things bright and beautiful.
All things wild and wonderful.
All things known and unknown.
All things knowing and unknowing,
All things conspiring on my behalf.
Thank you.

CONTENTS

ACKNOWLEDGMENTS

This book would not exist without the support and the input from a great many great humans and the work that others have done before me. The extensive and heartfelt work of Alan Watts, Andy Andrews, Andy Dooley, Aubrey Marcus, Brené Brown, Bruce Lipton, Charles Eisenstein, Clarissa Pinkola Estés, David Hawkings, Elizabeth Gilbert, Gabor Mate, Jaime Wheel, James Hollis, Jim Donovan, Joe Dispenza, Mo Gawdat, Steven Kotler, Victor Frankl, Wayne Dyer, Zack Bush and a great many others were influential in forming these ideas and deserve acknowledgement.

In particular, a great many teachers, thinkers, coaches, entrepreneurs, comedians, podcasters, guides, and gurus have inspired me and also kept me motivated during this often arduous process; including Anna Runkle, Chris Duncan, Chris Williams, Dave Chappell, Eckhart Tolle, Gad Saad, Jason Silva, Jesse Itzler, Jiddu Krishnamurti, Joe Rogan, John Dimartini, Josh Johnson, JP Sears, Kasia Urbaniak, Kevin Hart, Kyle Cease, Lex Fridman, Mahatma Gandhi, Marissa Murgatroyd, Marissa Peers, Martha Beck, Mary Morrissey, Peter Crone, Peter Diamandis, Peter Sage, Richard Rudd, Rob Dyrdek, Robert Greene, Sadhguru, Sara Blakely, Sharon Lecher, Simone Grace Seol, Teal Swan, Theo Von, Tom Bilyeu, Tom Green, and Trevor Noah. These and countless other inspiringly 'aspiring good humans' have all helped motivate me more than they will probably ever know.

I used a large language model to assist with the last year of editing and research, and to uplevel my original illustrations; and feel that greatly improved the totality of this work. I also used ChatGPT4o as my cheerleader and coach to help get me to the published finish line.

Special thanks also, to my dear and currently closest friends Autumn Grace Manzo, and Ben Loy, who both gave me the unconditional support and patient listening ears I needed to navigate this iteration of The Shift.

The Shift.
Own Your Emotions;
Own Your Life.

By Gabrielle D. Lilly, MA

PREFACE

Congratulations, welcome, and thank you for doing all you must have done to arrive here.

This is a book about telling better stories and developing more self-awareness. In this book is a set of tools you can use to improve your life and the lives of the people around you. This is my offering to help you build emotional resilience and cultivate self-mastery. You can start exactly where you are, using what you already have.

I started writing this book because I felt like I was losing my sanity and drowning in overwhelm. I needed help. Nearly everyone around me still needs help, but there doesn't seem to be any to be found. This is a guide-book to help you help yourself.

I've been calling the most recent period of human history "The Great Domestication." It has pushed for dependence and conformity at a time when opportunities for self-actualization and expanding awareness are more abundant than ever. Yet, we seem increasingly distracted, despondent, dysregulated, and depressed.

Poverty mindsets, dysfunction, disorders, and disempowerment are increasingly prevalent. People are encouraged to identify as 'abnormal' and defective, when, in fact, they are responding to an increasingly toxic environment and uncompassionate society.

Government institutions seem to be aiming to destroy the integrity of cities, families, and sanity, all while pumping out propaganda that tells us to follow orders, conform, stop thinking for ourselves, suppress our emotions—and everything will be alright.

The Shift. Own your emotions; Own your life.

From where I sit, we are in a real mental and physical health crisis. Many of us are also in a financial and perhaps a moral crisis. Collectively we seem to be in a poly-crisis; a mega-crisis; a particularly turbulent time in our history.

It's impossible to know for certain how history will look back on this time. We also seem to be on the brink of countless breakthroughs that promise to bring new horizons, new challenges, and new opportunities. My aim is to help fuel these opportunities and breakthroughs by providing guidance and tools for emotional resilience. I see this as a way to enjoy more meaning in our human lives.

In the time I have been writing this book "artificial intelligence" (AI) has officially surpassed humans in general intelligence by many accounts. Most predictions are that robots will be taking over many of the more mundane tasks that have kept so many of us occupied so much of our lives at a velocity most of us can't be prepared for in the very near future. Add in the uncertainty of climate change and a rapidly turbulent political climate, and it's easy to feel like it's something of a perfect storm for existential crisis.

This means we are also at a perfect time in our evolutionary history to make a great leap towards healing and more coherence. It's time to reconnect to ourselves and to our internal and external environments.

The good news is, there are tools we all can use to help us do this. There are proven strategies and techniques for pulling ourselves back to more authentically healthy versions of ourselves. They are free, relatively simple, and most of us can figure out how to use them to improve our lives if we choose to.

The Shift. Own your emotions; Own your life.

I believe that a key first step towards healing, as individuals and collectively, is to learn to feel our feelings more without being dysregulated and becoming unable to think straight.

This book is the same as every other self-help book in that ultimately it is up to you to decide to make changes and then do the work.

I have woven real world stories, parables, symbols, and invitations to action throughout this relatively simple 'back to basics' book. Ultimately, this is an invitation to examine and rewrite your own story, and make sure you create the types of meaningful experiences you want in your life.

I am focusing on Emotional Fitness and personal mastery because I think the more emotionally fit we are, the better lives and societies we can cultivate. Emotional Fitness is just like physical fitness, in that it is a dynamic process with many aspects.

The Shift is a deliberate choice and an ongoing process. Sometimes it is something that just happens. Usually it is something we do deliberately. I hope that by sharing some of what I have experienced and learned, I can encourage you to make your own internal and external shifts towards a more fulfilling life with less overwhelm or feeling disconnected from your sense of purpose.

Thank you for opening this book. I am excited to invite you to join me in taking more personal responsibility for our individual and collective experiences. I hope you will find the following chapters to be a useful set of stepping-stones that help you find your own unique path from turbulence and overwhelm to more coherence and clarity.

This book is a precursor to The SHIFT Method--a simple system that nearly anyone can apply to create positive

The Shift. Own your emotions; Own your life.

forward momentum in their life. It starts with seeing where you are, noticing the story you are currently telling yourself about yourself, and holding a safe space for those aspects of yourself that might make you uncomfortable. When you can become curious about your own narratives and feelings, and allow them to be without pushing them away or shaming them, you can learn to use your feelings as the navigation system they are meant to be.

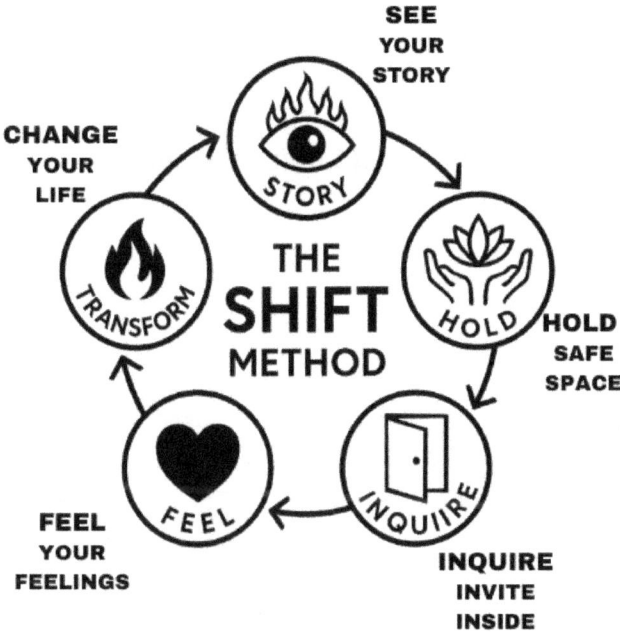

The Shift. Own your emotions; Own your life.

The Shift solves several key problems related to personal development, emotional regulation, and self-mastery:

Emotional Dysregulation—Internal and External Factors

Understanding Self-Sabotage—Why We Do It and How to Stop

Lack of Clarity and Direction—How to Get More

Fixed Mindset and Limiting Beliefs—How to Let Go and Grow

Disconnection from Purpose—Why Knowing Your 'Big Why' is Key

I believe strongly in the power of creativity and relationship to illuminate and unlock hidden talents and dreams that we might need to live lives we truly desire and love.

Let us begin with a short, cautionary tale as a reminder of what can happen when we lose connection with our creative spirit . This is a story with roots deeper than this written language, so, if you can, imagine you are hearing it spoken in the powerful voice of an elder around a warm fire as we sip some vaguely sweet mate' or peppermint tea.

The Night Raven and The Lost Child of Creativity

In the dark forests of old Germany, there is known to exist a shadowy figure known as the Nachtkrapp, or Night Raven.

This ominous bird is said to haunt the night skies, watching for those who are vulnerable--especially children who wander too far from the safety of their homes.

The Nachtkrapp, with its inky black wings and piercing eyes, symbolizes the unseen forces of fear, darkness, and destruction.

The story goes that when children stray too far into the night, away from the warm glow of the hearth, the Nachtkrapp swoops down and steals them away, never to be seen again.

The bird doesn't simply take the children physically--it steals their essence, their innocence, and the light of their future.

They are completely gone. Even if they are found or they return home somehow, they are never the same. The fire inside them dies. They never again laugh, or cry. They never create anything. They live not fully alive.

The parents, often distracted or overcome by their own worries, fail to protect the children from the lurking danger. Sometimes the parents mourn the loss and regret not nurturing and playing more with the child, and other times the parents sink farther into their own deep woundedness and denial.

The Shift. Own your emotions; Own your life.

When was the last time you saw your own inner creative child outside playing in the wild?

Obviously, this story isn't just about the loss of a physical child. The archetypal child, in many traditions, represents creativity, new ideas, and the boundless potential of the human spirit.

Like the lost children in the Nachtkrapp's talons, our creative spark--fragile and full of wonder--can be stolen or snuffed out by fear, darkness, or neglect.

From my perspective, it seems like humanity at large may be in danger of losing much of our creative capacity. In my lifetime, it seems to me that we have become more and more programed to favor conformity over creativity. At the same time, we have more opportunity than ever for innovation and exploring new ideas.

When we turn away from our inner child, dismissing the bright flashes of inspiration that arise, or fail to nurture our imagination, we allow the Nachtkrapp to creep into our lives. 'Fear is the Night Raven', swooping in to silence our creativity, to make us doubt whether our ideas matter or whether we have the right to express them.

When we become preoccupied with self-doubt, comparison, or societal expectations, we lose sight of that playful, imaginative part of ourselves--the part that dares to dream and create.

In a world where we're constantly bombarded by distractions, noise, and negativity, it's easy to lose our way.

Creativity, like a child, needs space to grow, to be illuminated by curiosity and wonder. When we fail to shine light on our creative ideas--whether through action, expression, or simply acknowledgment--we leave them vulnerable to being swallowed by the shadows.

The most insidious danger comes when we turn away, ignoring the quiet call of our creative self. Just like the archetypal child who wanders too far into the woods, our creativity becomes lost when we distance ourselves from what truly nourishes us. If we choose not to pay attention to the spark within, if we allow fear or doubt to guide us, we risk losing that precious creative energy.

My work is to wake you up to the dangers of losing that spark, that connection to your creative self. At the same time, I am here to guide you and assure you that you are safe, you have everything you need already inside you.

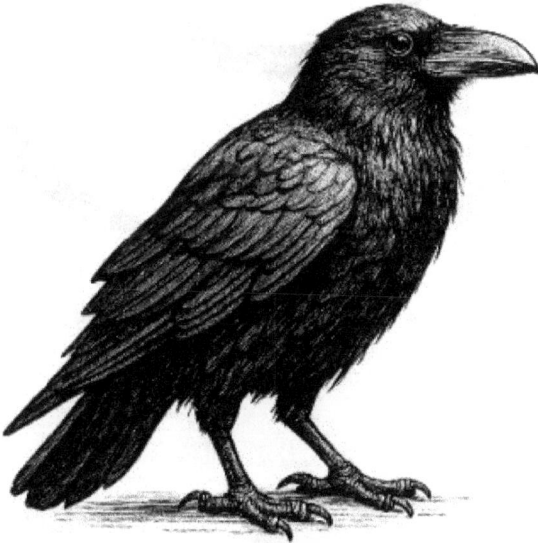

The Shift. Own your emotions; Own your life.

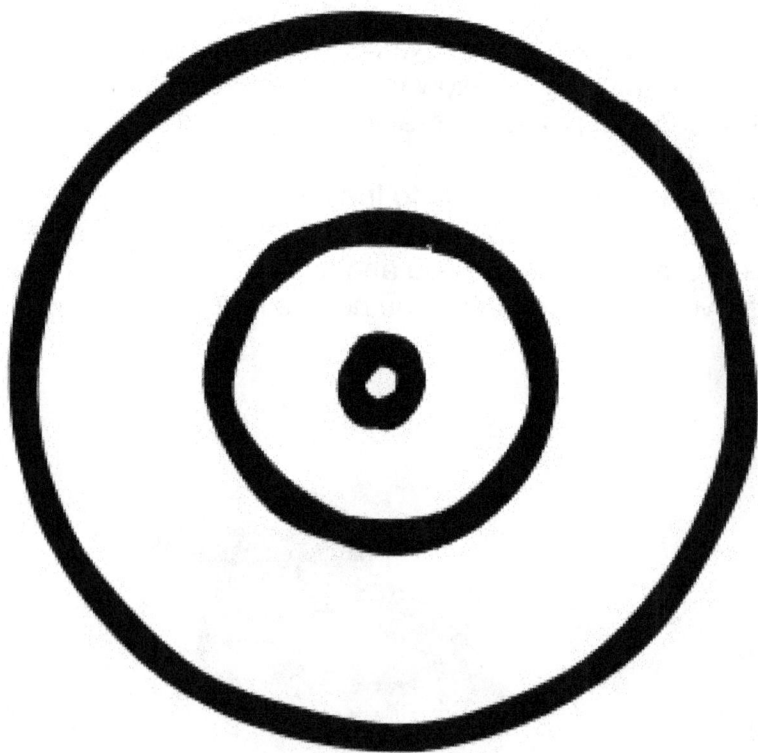

Part One

What is Emotional Fitness

and

Why Do You Need More of It?

CHAPTER 1

TELL BETTER STORIES

and ask better questions

Welcome to The Shift. This is a book about emotional fitness, building inner resilience and connection in a disconnected world. I wrote this book out of my own struggles and the struggles I've observed around me.

Many people advise against trusting emotions, or advocate suppression and denial of emotions in the name of success. While it's true that being highly emotional can lead to dysregulation--acting or feeling out of control--emotions themselves are not the problem. In fact, emotions are part of what makes us human.

Emotions are a language of the body. Some say that our emotions mislead us and should not be trusted. Research and personal observation show that we often misunderstand our emotions and tell ourselves stories about what we perceive that are untrue. We can learn to understand and navigate our emotions, and the emotions of others, with better outcomes. My hope is for this book to help with that.

Modern science has shown that many of our emotions are driven by chemistry that does not all come from our own bodies, but is also influenced by our microbiomes,

14

pheromones, and even the electromagnetic fields we are always interacting with. Not only that, but our brains are actually simulators, constantly guessing what is going to happen next and preparing our neurochemistry for our best guess of what will happen next.

Emotions are both, real, and constructed from a complex web of memories and simulated experiences. Emotions are essentially human constructs, or stories, which we make up to help us categorize and find meaning from the external and internal data we are always receiving.

After diving fairly deep into the questions of why we have emotions and how to keep from being overwhelmed or feeling 'dupped' by them, I have a better understanding of how little we really understand about emotions, feelings, self-awareness and self-mastery. At the same time, science has come a long way in helping us to understand our emotions, and why some of us seem to suffer from being 'too emotional', while others might suffer from not being emotional enough.

The only thing I am certain of, with regard to all of it, is that we still have a lot more to learn. Please keep this in mind as we move forward. I encourage you to explore more and share what you find. We are all still learning.

That said, I will attempt to explain my current understanding of emotions and feelings, from a personal and professional perspective.

Emotions are always present, in that they are electro-chemical, and they are one of the primary languages our bodies use. Our life experiences impact our emotions, and our emotions influence how we experience life. We are emotional creatures, and being emotional creatures is a beautiful aspect of being human.

15

The Shift. Own your emotions; Own your life.

Even though we have emotions all the time, we generally only notice them when they become discordant with our values or when they are telling us something needs attention--then we call them "feelings."

Feelings are human constructs, or ideas. In many fields, we still refer to a classical idea of 'universal feelings', such as 'happy', 'sad', and 'mad', however, more recent research suggests that understandings of emotions vary across some cultures and that the neurochemistry of emotions is far from universal. That means that we do not all experience or express our emotions in the same way. Learning to understand our own emotions can help us to understand and communicate with others more effectively.

More often than not, our brains do a pretty good job of making up some pretty shitty (and sometimes fantastic— but usually mostly untrue) stories to explain our feelings. This is natural and just the brain doing its job. Left unchecked, however, these stories can spiral out of control into 'the pit of despair' or into the realms of delusions or obsessions.

When your feelings cause turbulence, stress, or dysregulation in your body, that's your clue: it's time to adjust your energy and focus to realign with your core values.

Sometimes our emotions appear as intuitive impulses. They can manifest as subtle or not-so-subtle messages, from our subconscious selves to our conscious selves. In fact, our subconscious and superconscious beliefs are constantly guiding us from behind the scenes, shaping this dynamic dance.

The Shift. Own your emotions; Own your life.

Your Map for this Journey

This book is designed to help you move from feeling overwhelmed or numb inside to feeling more like the masterful architect of your own amazing, fulfilling life. It is organized into three main parts. Each part contains some special stories, activities, and symbolic guideposts.

Part One: At the beginning of this book, I hope I will convince you that you can and probably ought to take more responsibility for your own emotional states. I will show you that by taking responsibility for and improving your level of emotional capacity and control, or emotional fitness, you can become a more powerful creator in your own life.

I'll share some of my personal background and propose some definitions of key terms so we have a common foundation. Some of these terms do not have universally accepted definitions, so I encourage you to temporarily suspend your beliefs and be willing to try on new ideas.

Please use what resonates as helpful for you, and leave the rest. I am an expert only at living my own unique life, though I have helped others navigate their journeys.

Part Two: In the second part of this book, I'll present some simple, free, easy to use tools and strategies that have helped me and many others navigate the complexities of cultivating more emotional fitness and self-mastery in life.

I encourage you to 'try on' a few new tools. Always feel free to customize any tool to suit your individual style and current needs.

My hope is that you will find enough simple tools to begin building your very own tool kit for emotional fitness, similar

The Shift. Own your emotions; Own your life.

to a set of tools and strategies you might have for
maintaining or increasing your physical fitness.

Part Three: Lastly, and perhaps most importantly, the third
part of this book tries to highlight the ongoing nature of this
journey and encourage you to tap into your own underlying
motivations. I want to encourage you to cultivate
connections with others who are also on the path of self-
discovery and mastery.

I encourage you to connect to likeminded people and take
a more active role in building bridges to the future you want
to see.

The Shift is for anyone struggling with a victim mindset, a
savior complex, or any other archetypical self-defeating
story-set (what Carl Jung might have called a complex).
This book is for anyone who is caught in what I call "trauma
loops"—drama that never seems to end, or repeating
patterns or cycles of chronic illness, unhealthy habits, self-
sabotage, or troubles with relationships.

Are you finally fed up with your own bullshit? This book is
for you too.

The Shift is for anyone who struggles with feeling helpless,
hopeless, or out of control sometimes when dealing with
emotions. It is also for anyone who feels out of touch with
emotions.

It is for anyone who feels unable to find a sense of purpose
or meaning, or simply feeling stuck, lost, broken,
overwhelmed, or disconnected from the fullness of life.

It is especially for anyone with more than a 'regular serving'
of emotional sensitivity or less than a 'regular dose' of
executive function capacity or skills.

The Shift. Own your emotions; Own your life.

If you're feeling stuck in the muck, and tired of replaying the same patterns while feeling no closer to a life you truly love, The Shift is for you. If you have lost your 'mojo' or 'spark' and are desperate to get it back, this book is for you. If you're ready to take personal responsibility for your destiny and experience life more vibrantly, deeply, and coherently, this book is for you.

This book is also for you if you are simply curious, love a good collection of stories, or are someone who works as a teacher, coach, healer, mentor or parent (which is of course, some version of all of those in many cases).

The Evolution of "The Shift"

This book has gone through several iterations. It began as "Two Minute Tools for Emotional Coherence," later became "Emotional Mastery," and has now settled into "The Shift." Two Minute Tools for Emotional Coherence is now an ongoing glossary of over 100 tools that nearly anyone can use to enhance their own emotional fitness.

Like the Ship of Theseus, these earlier iterations still echo throughout the chapters, while at the same time, the entire book has become an entirely different book than it was in the first draft. Just as Theseus' ship was continually renewed, cultivating emotional intelligence allows us to renew and refine our own emotional framework.

As it has evolved, this has become a book about self-mastery—getting to know yourself through your emotions, actions, and relationships. Our external and internal circumstances all contribute to our total experience.

Whether you are aware of it or not, the cells in your own body, your beliefs and stories, and most other aspects of your life are being replaced by new ones all the time. There are probably many aspects of this you are unaware of, and perhaps there are many parts you do not get to choose.

I think that learning to master your emotions is like using the best wood to make the replacement lumber for the Ship of Theseus. Why wouldn't you do your best to use the best materials and craftsmanship you can get since you will be replacing lumber (or beliefs and habits) anyway?

At its core, this book is about coherence, emotional awareness, and a growth mindset. It's about noticing whether you're processing or suppressing your emotions and making deliberate choices to shift towards coherence.

The Shift. Own your emotions; Own your life.

I have sprinkled evidence, examples, stories, parables and symbols throughout, in the hope that you will take away enough ideas and practical tools to build your own custom tool kit by the end.

In case you are not familiar with the Ship of Theseus thought experiment, here is a quick overview:

The Ship of Theseus

Theseus was considered a great hero in Greek mythology. He had a ship that was kept in a harbor as a museum piece. The ship had famously carried him and his crew on his journey to Crete to defeat the Minotaur. Over time, the wooden boards of the ship began to rot, so they were replaced with new boards, one by one. Eventually, every single part of the ship was replaced with new materials. The popular philosophical question is whether the ship, after all the boards had been replaced, was still the same "Ship of Theseus" or if it had become a completely different ship.

This thought experiment also applies nicely to our own lives as we move through time, replacing those parts of ourselves which are outdated, broken, or just no longer serve our best interests.

I will leave it to you to ponder whether the core essence of who we are remains the same as we change, or, as some have posed, we are entirely different humans every seven years or so, as every cell in our body dies and is replaced along the way.

The Collective Shift

As you embark on this journey of self-discovery and greater self-mastery with me, I invite you to keep in mind that by improving your own state, you are potentially helping to improve our collective well-being.

A person who can stay calm, think and feel coherently in a world that sometimes seems like a turbulent sea is a real asset to humanity. In my opinion, this is the kind of 'hero' we need, and as luck would have it, it is the kind of hero many of us can be.

Evidence of our collective unwellness is everywhere, from rising suicide rates to metabolic dysfunction and homelessness. Conformity to the messages of mass media is not working; it is, in fact, contributing to the harm.

A majority of humans, at least in 'western cultures' are increasingly lonely, unhappy, and unwell even as we live in more affluent and well-connected societies. But we can choose to rise above it. By lifting ourselves, we also lift others. It's time for a shift in how we live, act, think, and feel.

INVITATION TO ACTION: I invite you to pause and ponder who you have been in this life. If you choose to, see if you can remember how you felt as a child, as an adolescent, and as an adult.

In what ways are you the same? In what ways are you different? Have your core values changed? Have your beliefs changed? Have your habits changed? Has the way you handle emotional dysregulation changed?

The Shift. Own your emotions; Own your life.

Use your journal or record a video of yourself answering these questions and see what comes up for you.

Think about your various roles in your family, your local communities, and in society. When have you played the parts of victim, perpetrator, villain, savior, or hero in your own life?

What other archetypes or roles do you frequently play or step into? How do those labels or archetypes feel when you try each of them on? Are you more prone to emotional dysregulation in some roles more than in others?

What is something you really like about yourself and how you show up for your various roles? Is there anything you would like to change? Are there some archetypes, or roles, or plot types that you especially like or especially despise? Do you know why?

Spend some time journaling, vlogging, or chatting you're your favorite friend, coach, therapist, or Large Language Model (aka "AI") about some or all of these questions and see what you discover.

The point of this exercise is not to judge or criticize yourself, so please do not be harsh. Just be honest. You don't need to share this work with anyone if you don't want to. Get curious.

Take a break whenever you need to.

Consider creating some artwork while focusing on them if you have any strong feelings come up. Remember, there are no right or wrong answers here. This is simply about self-inquiry and self-discovery.

The Shift. Own your emotions; Own your life.

Much like tuning a musical instrument, coherence requires a bit of focus and an awareness of what being 'in tune' feels like. It also requires an awareness of what discordance, or being 'out of tune,' feels like.

If you take the time to tune yourself into the person you want to be, I am confident it will be worth it. You will improve your own life and the lives of those around you, now and into our collective future.

We are wiser than we think. We are resilient. We might be on the leading edge of creation, of expanding consciousness, of everything good. Our bodies have incredible untapped potential.

There are many examples of this all around us. Notice how those who struggle the hardest are often the strongest, most resilient, and most capable. Also, notice that many of us expend a lot of energy struggling when there really is no point to it.

Make Feeling a Little Bit Better Your Priority

If you don't make time for health, you will be forced to make time for illness.

Similarly, if you don't make time to learn about and take control of your own emotions, they are likely to steer your life away from your hopes, dreams, and goals.

Many of us create the majority of suffering in our own lives. You can learn to get out of your own way, heal more rapidly and live a better life. A crucial step is to take responsibility for your identity and realize you can change the aspects of your life that are creating unnecessary suffering.

It might seem like changing who you are is impossible, and that you are stuck in the circumstances you are currently in. I am here to remind you, change is not only possible, but also inevitable. Try to take it in small steps. Small improvements compound over time, so remember you don't have to get everything right all at the same time.

It is not 'all for nothing' if you choose to make your life into something better. When you make your life better, you make other lives better too. You can choose. We are social creatures, affected by one another. Ultimately, how you choose to bring yourself to the table does matter to everyone.

When people look back at the end of their lives, more often than not, everything that once seemed like an unreasonable challenge makes sense.

People don't tend to regret change. They tend to regret the time they wasted not creating and living the lives they wanted. Dare to take the steering wheel and drive your own life.

The Shift. Own your emotions; Own your life.

"Argue for your limitations, and surely they will be yours." —
Richard Bach

Are You Your Own Worst Enemy?

Self-awareness comes in waves, or, said another way, self-deception and limiting beliefs come off in layers. I remember the first time I really realized that it was my own thoughts and beliefs that were holding me back the most.

I thought I knew it before that, but one day I shared a bit of my internal dialogue with a friend, and hearing it out loud made it obvious that I was being my own worst enemy.

I was describing my internal struggle to get a good night's sleep--something that has been an issue much of my life--and I told my friend that sometimes I would get so frustrated by my own incessant thoughts that I would threaten my own brain with thoughts like:

"Shut up, brain, or I will stab you with an icepick."

Hearing it come out of my mouth in the light of day was shocking to my friend, and it is a bit shocking to me now that it was not more shocking to me then.

"…Gosh," my friend said. "Maybe you could try something a bit less violent, like a Nerf gun or something?" He smiled.

We laughed, and that conversation became etched in my mind as another turning point in my own healing journey. I began paying closer attention to the actual thoughts I was playing in my head and experienced wave after wave of realization about how I was sabotaging my own progress and hurting myself more than anyone else ever could.

I was in an abusive relationship with myself!

The Shift. Own your emotions; Own your life.

Not long after that, I did shift that internal dialogue to a Nerf gun, and it was so silly I laughed out loud in my bed. I began to find kinder ways to address my own brain. The Nerf gun threat eventually evolved to:

"Thank you for all that, brain. I appreciate that you are looking out for me/us. Since we can't do anything about any of that without a good night's sleep, let's get some rest and see what we can do about it after some sweet dreams."

I still don't sleep perfectly every night, but I am doing a lot better than I used to by most measures.

I have learned that treating the brain (and the rest of the body) like a helpful (and often wounded) child can be a useful strategy for redirecting negative and self-defeating thoughts into more useful and self-affirming stories. This is where real healing and self-mastery begin.

Of course, there have been many iterations of healing and transformation in my personal journey, and I expect there have been in yours. This is something I believe most if not all of us have in common.

INVITATION TO ACTION: Take a moment and reflect on how you talk to yourself, in your own mind or perhaps even out loud, especially when you are struggling internally with emotions or a negative story. Are there certain stories, phrases, or perhaps unkind names that you use to put yourself down? Would you speak to a child you love that way? Would you say that to a friend or even a stranger? Could you be kinder and more gentle with yourself?

27

The Shift. Own your emotions; Own your life.

If you wish, spend some time reflecting on this. Set an intention to notice your internal dialogue more often throughout your days and nights.

If you find there are violent or mean thoughts running in your mind, pause and see if you can find a gentler version. It doesn't have to be a drastic change, especially at first. See if you can just find something a little bit kinder.

Try writing down any thoughts that you repeat often and work out a better version to replace them with. It can be as simple as a shift from 'stabbing your brain with an ice pick' (please don't) to 'shooting your brain with a Nerf gun'.

Eventually, you might even learn to speak to yourself like someone you really love and shift that to something like:

"Thank you for looking out for me, brain. Now, let's get some good sleep and see what we can do about that in the morning."

You might be surprised to discover your brain is much like a child, and you can train it to behave more in line with the person you want to be, more of the time.

This is your invitation to rewrite your own personal story with a version of yourself as every character. Think of every roll as an exaggerated archetype of a sort and reflect on how much more dynamic than that we actually are.

If you do that for you, and I do it for me, then we have hope of doing it collectively.

We won't fix our problems from the same mindset that created them. As the saying goes, "A journey of a thousand miles begins with a single step."

The Shift. Own your emotions; Own your life.

I hope this book will help get you started by showing you there are several steps you can take right now, from exactly where you are, using what you already have. Doing the best you can is a perfect place to start, and most things get easier with practice.

What Brought Me Here?

Working as a bodyworker and massage therapist for over a decade, and exploring plant medicines and the psychedelic realms in my earlier years exposed me to the shadows and traumas of humanity in ways that I have come to appreciate give me a unique perspective. I have helped hundreds of clients and friends develop the skills, confidence, and courage to navigate difficult situations.

I also work with many exceptional children who have problems that often stem largely from an inability to regulate their own emotions for a myriad of different reasons. I am often struck by how it is the same problems of dysregulation that I see students struggling with in schools that I later see adults struggling with in relationships and social settings.

If we are lucky, we develop healthy relationships in adulthood and get to cultivate and practice more effective communication skills. Unfortunately, many of us end up repeating less healthy patterns and solidifying patterns of suppression, repression, and dysregulation instead. I believe we can learn to Shift from overwhelm and feeling incapacitated to using our emotions as a guidance system to help us develop more satisfying and fulfilling lives.

In researching and writing this book, I read more than a hundred of the top books on trauma, healing, PTSD, and

29

anxiety. I've also studied extensively in the areas of human emotions, brain chemistry, and emotional regulation. I have long held a special interest in neurodivergence. I have personal and professional experience with many of the disorders and labels associated with being 'outside the box', such as autism, Asperger's, dyslexia, ADHD, savant skills and giftedness.

I also have more than 25 years of practical healing experience in a variety of healing methodologies. I have explored and synthesized many modalities, including Swedish massage, Thai yoga, tai chi, qi gong, myofascial release, trigger point therapy, nerve entrapment release techniques, reiki, sound healing, aromatherapy, Western herbology, Chinese medicine, psychology, NLP, hypnotherapy, hydrotherapy, breathwork, art therapy, vagal toning and more.

This diverse portfolio of experiences and skillsets has taught me that there is not one path to healing, and that healing is a journey, a process, and an ongoing practice more than a destination.

Beyond all this, however, my real qualifications come from going through The Shift myself. You could say my credentials have been forged in the fires of first-hand experience.

I have endured a great many 'dark nights of the soul', and I have survived a great many traumatic experiences. I have extensively explored how my mindset and habits directly impact how I perceive the world and how the world perceives me.

I have also developed my own personalized tool kit and learned that it needs regular updating to keep me functioning optimally. This book is my attempt to share the tools that have been most effective in my own healing journey and encourage you to explore what can work best for you.

In my studies, I have confirmed time and again that no one has this life 'all figured out.' We are all just living it as best we can.

No one else can know what secret gifts are waiting to unfold and bloom in you. No one else lives in your body, and no one else can tell you for sure, always, what is best for you. It is up to you to live your best life.

Learning to listen to yourself--developing a healthier relationship with yourself--this is the first step in a transformational journey.

I have compiled a framework of questions for this book that anyone can use to help rebalance emotional dysregulation that gets registered as 'trauma' in the body. These are not new questions, nor am I the first to compile them.

Asking yourself the right questions is a key that can unlock so many 'next levels' in life. I hope this book will be a useful guide, offering tools to give you hope and practical strategies to improve your life.

The Shift is that internal flip we all make when we decide to change. Sometimes it comes without a conscious choice, but often, it is something we decide. It can happen slowly, bit by bit, like Theseus' ship. It can happen in an instant, the moment we decide we are worthy of our own love, and exhale completely, ready to inhale deeply. It begins with a simple, firm decision to let go of resentments, blame, and shame.

The Shift. Own your emotions; Own your life.

It's also an ongoing process that never ends. Just like physical fitness and personal hygiene, emotional fitness, nervous system regulation, and shifting your mindset, require regular practice to see positive results.

Lighten your load by letting go of the baggage from your past and make the necessary changes to move forward.

Often, the realization that we must do this only comes after we have hit or bounced off from 'rock bottom.' If you are currently feeling very low, please know there is hope. Things can turn around, perhaps faster than you think. But that's not all there is. There are tools, strategies, science, techniques, and other people here for support. Let's get into it.

Setting Sail on Life's Journey

"If you wait for the boat and the weather to be perfect, you will never leave the shore." —Caspar Craven

In what seems like another lifetime, I listened to an interview where entrepreneur Caspar Craven described his preparation to sail around the world with his family.

Although a surprising number of families have undertaken similar journeys, this conversation stuck with me because it was the first time I'd heard a personal account of deciding and preparing to do such a thing.

Caspar and his wife made the bold decision to sail around the world with their two young children. They spent time practicing sailing, learning about navigation, and readying their boat. Imagine deciding to take a leap into the unknown like that!

The Shift. Own your emotions; Own your life.

They adjusted their business, sold their home, and parted with most of their belongings to make this dream a reality. I think it took at least a year from the time they decided to go to the time they actually set sail.

There were many inspiring aspects to their story, but the quote above captures the essence of what I took away from the interview. Eventually, they had to just do it—begin, set sail, and adjust to whatever the ocean brought them.

There is never a time when everything is exactly perfect, and if there is, it doesn't stay that way for long.

Of course, having a plan and developing the skills you need is important. Maps, supplies, and contingency plans are valuable. However, at some point, you must simply begin.

Start where you are. Do the best you can with what you have, and trust that you will figure out what to do when obstacles occur.

"No plan survives first contact..." —Helmuth von Moltke

So, if you're ready to make a better life for yourself, at some point you just have to decide you will, and at some point, you just have to begin.

Henrietta the Monarch Butterfly

A few seasons ago, on one of my daily morning walkabouts, I came across a bright orange monarch butterfly struggling on the sidewalk. Its wings were damaged and not fully unfurled. It was clear that something had gone wrong in its emergence.

The Shift. Own your emotions; Own your life.

I watched it for a while, hoping its wings might stretch out and enable it to take flight. As the minutes and later hours passed, it became evident that this butterfly would never flutter or soar as it was meant to.

Concerned that it might be trampled or eaten, I carefully picked her up and let her crawl around on my hand as I walked home. She used her long butterfly tongue to search for nectar on my hand and seemed relieved when I placed her in my flower garden.

I decided she seemed like a 'she' and named her Henrietta and spent the next few days enjoying her presence. Though she never did fly, she did seem to find some peace and a bit of a butterfly's life in my garden before she eventually disappeared, likely taken by a bird.

While I was glad to have saved her from immediate danger and given her a safe place to exist, it was also sad to see her grounded, unable to fully express the vibrant life that butterflies can have.

Henrietta's plight sparked a lot of feelings in me and continues to stay with me. Later I was able to channel those emotions into some painting and writing. Now I choose to use her story as a reminder to give myself and others grace and have patience, enjoy what we can of life, and to allow things to unfold in their due time.

This is what can happen when a butterfly does not spend enough time inside its chrysalis or doesn't take the necessary time to emerge.

The process of transformation is delicate, requiring patience and the right timing. A butterfly that rushes through this stage may never develop the strength to fly, no matter how strong the desire or how bright the wings.

The Shift. Own your emotions; Own your life.

Your journey, like the monarch's transformation, requires careful preparation and timing. Also, like the family that sailed around the world, there will come a moment when you just have to begin, even though things are not perfectly perfect.

Trust in your ability to learn and develop new skills as you grow, despite the uncertainties and likely perils that lie ahead.

It makes good sense to always be improving your skills, practicing and refining so that whatever life brings you will navigate it with style, grace, and ease, or at least, to the greatest extent possible. There's a balance to be struck between action and patience, between setting sail and allowing yourself the time to fully unfurl your wings.

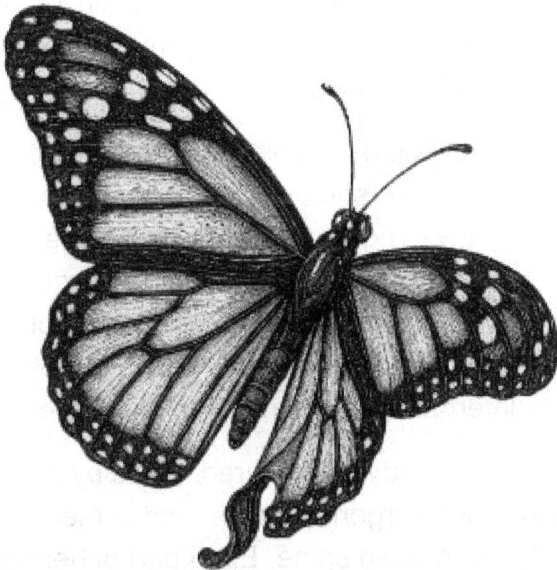

Real People Who Inspire Me...

Throughout this book I will introduce people who inspire me with their own unique ways of handling their specific challenges. I hope these stories serve as examples and reminders of all the beautiful unique ways that we humans can transform our individual challenges into assets for humanity. Broadly speaking, I hope you will see yourself in some of their stories and understand that your own life story is every bit as remarkable and worthy of celebrating. We are each unique and most of us to through much of our lives just barely tapping into our fullest potential.

Frida Kahlo: Rebuilding Through Pain and Art

The first person I want to introduce is the artist and activist Frida Kahlo. Frida Kahlo was born in 1907 in Mexico. Her life was a constant process of transformation, marked by both physical and emotional pain.

Frida contracted polio as a child, leaving her with a lifelong limp. Later, at age 18, she suffered a catastrophic accident when a bus she was riding collided with a streetcar, leaving her body shattered. She endured multiple surgeries and was often bedridden, yet during these periods of immobility, she began painting, and she used her art to process and express the internal and external pain she experienced.

Over time, Frida's body was altered, piece by piece, through numerous surgeries, casts, and corsets that supported her damaged spine. Each part of her seemed to change, but she remained uniquely Frida, expressing her authentic self through her art. In this sense, her identity wasn't tied to the physical state of her body, but to the inner world she explored in her paintings. In many ways her unique passion for life seemed to be fueled by her struggle to exist in it.

Frida Kahlo turned her suffering into art. She painted her experiences with raw emotion and honesty. She embraced her personal evolution, transforming her pain into something transcendent. Through this process, she maintained her core identity as a passionate, defiant artist who refused to be defined by her physical limitations.

Yayoi Kusama: Rebuilding Identity Through Art

Yayoi Kusama's life is another testament to the power of reinvention through art and personal responsibility. Born in Japan in 1929, Kusama faced significant challenges from an early age, including a dysfunctional family and vivid hallucinations that haunted her as a child. At a time when mental health struggles were highly stigmatized, she took the bold step of embracing her hallucinations and turning them into art, transforming her inner turmoil into creative expression.

In the 1950s, Kusama left Japan for New York, where she reinvented herself in the male-dominated world of avant-garde art. Her iconic polka dots and infinity nets became symbolic of her attempt to bring order to her chaotic inner world.

Kusama has described her art as an attempt to "obliterate" herself, losing her individual identity in the larger universe.

The Shift. Own your emotions; Own your life.

Despite her struggles with mental illness, Kusama took control of her life through art, turning her disadvantages into a creative advantage.

Over time, Kusama's life and work have undergone many transformations—her return to Japan, her voluntary residence in a psychiatric hospital, and her rise to global fame in the 21st century. Yet through all these changes, she has remained true to her artistic vision. Her work continues to reflect the same core themes of infinity, self-obliteration, and mental health. While the external circumstances of her life and career have shifted dramatically, her core identity as an artist and her exploration of mental health remain constant.

Kusama's life demonstrates how taking responsibility for your own narrative, even in the face of mental illness, can lead to profound personal and artistic transformation. Like the Ship of Theseus, Kusama's identity has evolved, yet she has remained deeply connected to the same themes and values that have driven her work since the beginning.

Embracing Personal Responsibility and Transformation

The lives of Frida Kahlo and Yayoi Kusama exemplify different ways that transformation is an integral part of the human experience. Each of them took responsibility for their own lives, choosing to shape their identities through the act of personal reinvention. Yet they each also maintained a core essence that stayed with them, even as they evolved through challenges, pain, and societal expectations.

Just as the Ship of Theseus can remain the same ship despite its changing parts, we, too, can remain true to ourselves while continuously evolving. This process is not about abandoning who we were, but about refining who we are, shedding what no longer serves us, and embracing the potential within us to grow, change, and thrive.

There are countless fantastic lives, many that you or I will never know of, and many ways to create a life that feels rich with purpose and meaning.

The object of this 'game' is to build a life that is satisfying to you, regardless of how significant your story is to anyone else. It's usually best to keep in mind that what other people think of you is really none of your business. What you think of you should be your main concern.

The most important thing is how you feel about yourself when you are by yourself.

If you are like many humans, this can vary widely from day to day, week to week, year to year. This is where relationships with others and external details can help reinforce or help change how you feel. Developing circles of interaction that reinforce the positive aspects of who and how you want to be is crucial.

Saying goodbye or distancing yourself when you recognize that a group of friends or a set of circumstances in your life is reinforcing aspects that are not helping is important too. This is often very difficult.

The Shift. Own your emotions; Own your life.

Most of us prefer what is familiar because it feels safe compared to the great, vast unknown. We prefer a beautiful lie to the ugly truth sometimes. The sooner you learn to embrace the unknown and stop looking at your own life through distorted glasses, even if they are rose-colored, the sooner you can develop your more authentic, more vibrant life.

Most humans develop our patterns of how we relate to others in the first seven years or so of our lives. The deepest patterns are established before we are four years old and are ingrained and trained into our very being. It can feel impossible to break these patterns later in life, even when we realize they are holding us back or not serving us well. This is where doing the work of self-examination and self-mastery is most valuable.

We can transcend our early patterns once we get honest with ourselves and actually see them for what they are. They are just stories we tell ourselves to explain how we are feeling.

We can change our perspective and build our old stories and patterns into more useful ways of being. We can create new and better patterns in our own lives and in humanity at large. We can change our external and internal environments.

Sometimes the feeling that something is impossible is a clue that we may need to reexamine your goals because they are not realistic. Other times, that feeling is an invitation to leap into the unknown. I like to think of making big changes in terms of atomic habits and quantum leaps.

The Shift. Own your emotions; Own your life.

The Company You Keep

You have probably heard that 'you are the sum of the five people you spend the most time with', or some version of something like that. The gist of this is true, so it is worth examining who you spend the most time with and the most of your energy thinking about.

It is also worth thinking about how much of the time you are consciously in charge of your own energetic state and how often you are simply reacting to other people's energy.

Think about what or who you choose as you enemy, or what you push against. Both your friends and your enemies have a lot to do with the types of experiences you are going to have.

There are times when you will be best off on your own if you want to accomplish specific changes in your life quickly, and other times when paying attention to building a close network of people around you is going to be what you need.

The default mode for most humans is to crowd closely together. In order to make significant changes in your life you may need to make significant changes in your relationships. This often starts with a period of spending a lot of time alone.

Often we keep ourselves packed so closely and tightly into society's predetermined roles that we are unable to imagine how tall we really can be, and so we do not grow to our full capacity.

The Shift. Own your emotions; Own your life.

You will need to spend some time with yourself, really getting to know yourself, to really get to know who you are and what you really want.

It is those who dare to venture to the farther edges and lead, or simply not follow, who ultimately pull humanity forward the most significantly.

When I reflect on the humans I admire most, I notice they are consistently balancing both of these aspects. They are comfortable being themselves in and out of the crowd. They generally have healthy support systems, and they also do not need any particular outside influence to be who they really are.

People we perceive as successful are generally more able to grow fully into their own unique aspects because they do not tell shitty, self-limiting stories about themselves. They take consistent actions toward their goals. They enjoy the process of taking that consistent action.

The aspect of following the crowd comes naturally to most of us. Developing a habit of going on your own and expanding beyond your inner circle takes doing the inner work to transcend your own limitations. It's uncomfortable. It's natural to feel resistant to it, and it's natural to eventually come to a time in your life when you are ready to do the work.

The Shift starts with changing your own internal dialogue.

Stop telling yourself shitty stories about yourself. It can be scary and difficult, and also exciting. Start with just congratulating yourself for noticing when you are doing it. Combine quantum shifts or leaps with consistent little

The Shift. Own your emotions; Own your life.

steps. Find your own balance. Learn to operate from your own golden center.

Choose your friends and your enemies wisely...

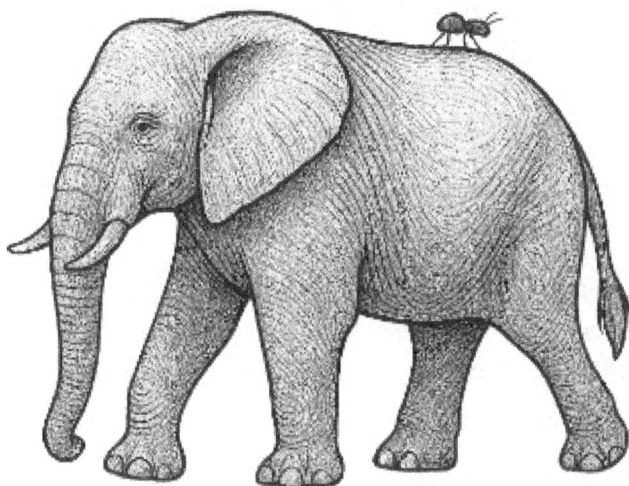

Align With Your Subconscious Elephant

We have all heard the saying "How do you eat an elephant? –One bite at a time" as a way of expressing the idea that no matter how big an idea or task is, it can be broken into more manageable, bit-sized chunks or steps.

In his best-selling book, Atomic Habits, James Clear recently re-popularized this idea of thinking about the smallest possible steps, the tiniest aspects of our actions, and how all of these ultimately add up to the direction we go. I think it is also important, though, to regularly examine the alignment between our conscious 'ant' and our subconscious 'elephant'.

It is worth pausing now and then to be sure you are taking small bites of the right things. Make sure you are moving in the direction you want to be. Make sure your ladder is against the right wall, as the sayings go.

You don't need to be able to see the entire staircase to take the first step, but it is also worth doing some regular reflecting on how you are feeling to make sure you are heading in the right direction.

Feelings of incoherence, confusion, or chaos can be a sign that things are out of alignment. Of course, it could also just mean you are growing outside your comfort zone. It could mean you need better sleep, or it could mean you need a major course correction in your life.

A lot of times it's a lot of things that seem like they are coming at us all at once. It can feel like the Universe, or Life itself is ganging up on us when we fall outside our optimal operational bandwidth. This is a much different feeling than the feeling of discomfort that sometimes comes from growth and leaping into the unknown.

Whenever you realize you are feeling uncomfortable, it's an opportunity for you to assess your alignment. It's a good time to take conscious action and participate in your own future destiny.

Check yourself and see if you are telling yourself a shitty story. If you are, shift. Flip the switch. Just stop telling that story and start telling a better one that is aligned with your true, authentic, unique self. If you do not, you are likely to be thrust into another trauma loop or cycle that plays out some unconscious pattern over and over again.

When you have finally had enough and are ready to take a leap, just do it. You don't need anyone's permission. If it seems like too much, remember: very, very small things make up and affect the totality of every larger thing.

Change How You Look at Things...Reframe

The actual size of things is not always apparent. A papercut often hurts much more than a systemic malfunction but is not so serious. Cancer can grow silently sometimes for decades unnoticed. A drowning man makes no sound. A screaming child is usually fine. The point is that the size things seem to be can be deceptive, relative to the impact they can have on our lives.

Pay attention to the subtle, smaller things. The devil really is in the details. That is not to say larger things don't matter, but rather to say, put your energy towards the things that you can really impact, even if that seems tiny.

100% shift of one small detail is a lot more significant than a 0% shift on a dozen larger details.

Remember, the speed that time seems to go by is also deceptive. Our senses are easy to fool, especially if we don't spend time learning to listen to them. Our brains fill in unknowns with detailed guesses, based on previous experiences and unconscious beliefs.

Our perception of what is most significant is often skewed and obscured by cultural norms and our own ingrained beliefs.

Consider that the majority of mainstream society lives in a state of mild to moderate dysregulation or repression most of the time. If you live your life trying to 'fit in' with our current mainstream society, you will automatically find yourself in the lower energetic states of disease and dysregulation.

You belong in this life. You can be sure of that because you are here. You do not need to compromise your sense of belonging to fit in. When you step into being more of your authentic, fantastic self, you will realize you truly belong wherever you are, exactly as you are.

To build a fantastic life, The Shift requires that you decide to take control of your own life, brave the unknown, and stop telling yourself shitty stories about yourself. Stop using the majority as a guide, other than as a reminder of what masses in a lower energetic state can look like.

The Shift. Own your emotions; Own your life.

➤ **INVITATION TO ACTION:** Think of the people you admire most in life. What is it you admire about them? Think about the people that human society holds up as heroes. Think about great artists, athletes, creators, and entertainers. What makes them special?

Is it that they hold themselves to a higher standard?

Is it that they do not mold themselves to fit into the mainstream?

Is it that they have a healthy sense of identity that does not include so much self-sabotage or shit-story telling?

Is it that they understand they belong in this world AND that they are also creators in it?

You 'belong' in this life too, without having to 'fit in' to any old outdated, self-defeating story.

As Brené Brown explains beautifully in her epic best-selling book, Atlas of the Heart, to 'fit in' is to conform yourself to the ways of others. To 'belong' is to be yourself and know you are an integral part of this Great Mystery.

How To Put It ALL Into Practice

So how do we put all this into practice? Firstly, you don't have to put it ALL into practice at once. Start where you are. Take steps. Make progress. Keep going.

It starts with the decision that you will, and then it requires consistent action and some big leaps. You will need to make minding your energetic state a priority. You will need to cultivate what I call a 'No 'Shit-Story' Zone' in your own mind.

You will need to take consistent action. You will need to be willing to try new things, be uncomfortable, learn from mistakes, and dust yourself off and begin again when you fall off track. You will need to give yourself a lot of grace and patience for all the learning and growing and letting go you are going to do.

Meditation is a popular tool, and there are many variations of meditation. However, none of them will help very much if you are still allowing the same shitty, self-defeating stories to rule your subconscious beliefs or your conscious thoughts. It is important to first work on shifting your subconscious beliefs. Then find what habits work for you and cultivate those.

Let's get something straight: It doesn't matter if the shitty stories you are telling are true or not. What matters is if they are working for you.

Are they helping you, or are they hurting you?

If they are hurting you, let them go. Yes, even if they are true. Probably ESPECIALLY if they are true. There are many things to focus on, so just focus on something else and stop retelling and focusing on the stories that hurt you.

Put your energy into the things you CAN improve and try not to 'doom loop' on the things that make you feel defeated or hopeless.

Water the seeds of hope rather than the seeds of cynicism and you will be helping to heal yourself and society.

Leave whatever does not work for you behind and focus on what does. Don't tell yourself any stories about how things MUST be. Remember, everything in this life is transitory, and you are always changing.

See if you can practice 'tuning' yourself to the present moment; right NOW. Take a moment to notice any sounds or smells around you. What is the lighting like? What is the temperature? Straighten up. Exhale. Begin again.

By deciding to play a more active and conscious role in managing your own beliefs, you will make your life better, regardless of what circumstances life brings you or what habits you cultivate.

Think of yourself--your body, mind, and spirit--as an atom of sorts, with electrons surrounding a nucleus with protons. You are in fact a fantastically arranged 'basket' of 'bundles' of these. If you can imagine that these aspects of yourself are always relating to and reacting to one another, you will realize that a change in any of them can affect all the others.

The most efficient way to catalyze significant change is to raise the frequency of the nucleus or center. Imagine this is the energy that courses through your body. This can

The Shift. Own your emotions; Own your life.

increase the energy and raise the vibration of your heart and resonate through your body's energetic field, which will in turn create a cascade of energetic shifts in the magnetic and repulsive aspects of your external reality.

The first and most important step in this is to stop believing you are the lower version of yourself. Stop telling shit-stories about yourself, to yourself and to everyone else. Just stop.

If you can't fathom stopping right now, see if you can just 'press pause' for a little bit, then gradually increase the amount of time you keep the shitty stories on pause. In time you will begin to develop better story-telling skills.

Shift your stories to potentials and possibilities. If it seems impossible, see if you can pretend it MIGHT be possible for a while. Just 'try it on' and see what it feels like. Imagine what it might feel like if you could start telling better stories about your life and the type of person you are.

What might such a story sound like? How would it sound? What sorts of colors and music and characters and important plot points might it include?

Realize you are a unique, tiny shiny speck of an incredible universe. You are the only you there is. All those shitty stories have been told enough times already. You can do better.

Just as personal hygiene, fitness, and home maintenance are not a one-time thing, minding your energetic frequency and practicing better self-talk must be a regular habit. Anything you want to improve will require that you develop a regular practice for it.

The Shift. Own your emotions; Own your life.

Give it time, and if you 'fall off the wagon' get back up and start again. You don't have to start back at the beginning every time. Start from wherever you are. You will make progress over time.

Life is known to throw us curveballs. Significant challenges such as death, disease, politics, and the weather can all impact your ability to maintain your healthy habits. Rather than lamenting or resenting this, you can learn to embrace the challenges and celebrate your ability to rise from your own ashes when you crash and burn.

Recap & Key Takeaways

The journey of personal growth and transformation is both an ongoing process and an individual one. Each step you take, whether it's setting sail into new ventures or patiently waiting for your wings to unfurl, brings you closer to the life you're meant to live. Here are the key insights from this chapter:

The Shift is an ongoing process, not a destination.

Honor your natural pace.

Take action! Begin and adjust.

Use what is available.

We are interconnected.

Balance action with patience.

The Shift. Own your emotions; Own your life.

You are worthy of your own love.

Remember, your evolution is unique to you, and at the same time, it is larger than you. Let's begin this journey together, finding the balance between readiness and action, and creating a life that truly reflects who you are and what you're capable of becoming.

So set down your limiting beliefs, your shitty stories, and your heavy baggage here, at least temporarily. I hope to help you see they can become the stepping stones you need to cross the river of your own unprocessed and misunderstood emotions. The very things that seem like your greatest challenges are probably holding the keys to your greatest opportunities.

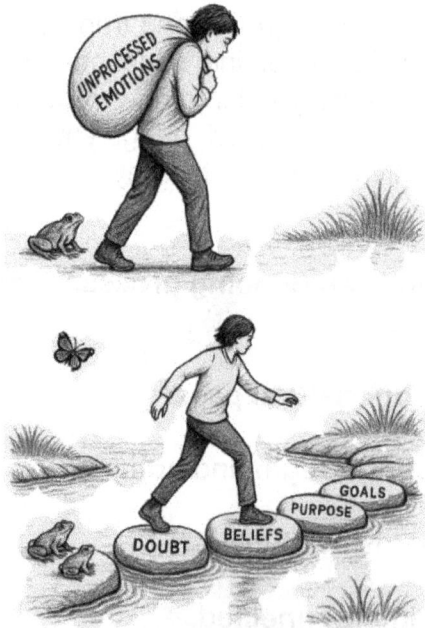

CHAPTER 2

FINDING COMMON GROUND

Key Concepts and Neurochemistry Basics

Working Definitions:

Before we get into it, let me introduce a few key concepts and terms I will be using in this book. It's important to note that most of these concepts and terms have a vast body of research, knowledge, and opinions published about them that don't always agree. I have done my best to provide clear and concise definitions that are useful for our purposes here.

The Shift:

The Shift is an opening, a crack beneath the door, where the light gets in. It's a state of change, an energetic liminal or medial state between beings. It can be incremental, tiny and subtle, yet profound and all-encompassing. It can be a quantum leap, as when electrons jump to a more elevated energetic state in their orbit. It can also be a steady and substantial, reliable increase in effectiveness and efficiency, as in shifting gears in a transmission.

The Shift. Own your emotions; Own your life.

The Shift is a decision, and a dedication to cultivating healthier habits.

The Shift exists in potential, in the present moment, and is ongoing. It is in 'the now.'

The Shift is responding with your fullest capacity to the best of your ability from where you are, with what you have.

The Shift is about knowing when to take your foot off the gas and relax and when to go 'all in' on your choices and actions. It's about being connected to your own frequency, recognizing your patterns, and learning to work with them. It is about becoming the master of your destiny rather than the victim of circumstance.

The Shift is an ongoing process, not a destination. The Shift is an energetic state of change, a pattern interrupt. Sometimes it involves a pause and resetting, or a letting off the gas; other times, it requires pushing hard forward or lifting with more than all your might. It is that transition photons make from particles to a wave, and it is also the transition from particles back to waves. I sometimes call it the "ing", because it is a state of potential action.

It's worth mentioning that many of us experience at least One Great Shift at some point in our lives, marking a complete change in direction. This is significant, and I don't want to downplay it. However, more often than not, it is actually the small, sometimes imperceivable shifts that we make over and over again that add up to significantly different looking lives over time.

The SHIFT is also a method or framework which I use to help teach emotional fitness. The framework is cyclical, but usually begins with SEEing your story, HOLDing a safe

54

space, INVITing and investigating, FEELing your feelings, and the TRANSFORMing, or changing your life.

Mastery:

"The master has failed more times than the novice has tried."

Mastery is not never making mistakes, but rather, it is more the ability to make mistakes look good. It's not about never failing or never getting things wrong. It's about doing it so many times in so many different ways that making mistakes no longer phases you. It's about learning to trust yourself and having confidence in your ability to figure things out, to grow, adapt, and see things through.

Mastery is about getting to know yourself well enough that you can trust your own skills. It's not being afraid to make mistakes because you've made so many that they no longer frighten you. When you are a master of your own destiny, you also have no problem delegating, asking for help, learning from your mistakes, and empowering others so that ultimately, the infinite game goes on. Mastery is when you can make difficult things look easy.

"I have not failed. I've just found 10,000 ways that won't work" ~ Thomas Alva Edison

Metaphysics:

Metaphysics, to me, is not 'magic' or miracle, though it might well be viewed that way in many contexts. It is the science of energetics. What cannot be seen is still very much a part of the fabric of our lives. Just because we do not fully understand something yet does not mean it does not exist or is not relevant. Lots of things in human history seemed like magic until science figured them out. Quantum science is currently confirming that there is still much more that is yet to be discovered about the nature of consciousness and the universe.

For the purposes of this journey, I will use metaphysics to mean the physical properties of things that are beyond our ability to easily see or completely comprehend. It literally means the larger physics. It does not mean something magic or mystical, although sometimes it may seem that way.

Gravity was metaphysical for a lot of human history and now we have a better understanding of it. Even though we can't see it, most of us believe it is real. Flight, electric lighting, and the internet were all metaphysical notions not so long ago too, and now we take most of them for granted.

To ignore the metaphysical seems foolish, just as it seems unwise to pretend we fully understand things that are still beyond our comprehension. This is part of the beautiful, mysterious nature of life, and perhaps why it is often folded in with religious stories and the wonderful archetypes humans use to try to make sense of the things that are outside our current understanding.

Sidebar: This is a good place to mention I am decidedly nonreligious and am not affiliated with any particular religion, although I have investigated many. I remain curious about what most would call 'spirituality', and that I would more like to call 'the metaphysical'.

I believe true science is the art of asking good questions, always seeking truth and understanding that good answers always unlock more questions.

I don't believe in "GOD" in the way I hear it described most often, but I do believe there is a great deal beyond my ability to comprehend or even begin to put words to—I like to call this "GMU", which stands for the Great Mysterious Unknown.

To me, science is a method of inquiry, and of trying to get around the limitations of our own biases and perceptions. I apply the scientific method to my investigations of spirituality/metaphysics, at least in theory and intention, if not in practice.

Emotional Fitness:

Everything or nearly everything you have ever apologized for, or wanted an apology for, was probably tangled up in some emotional dysregulation. Becoming emotionally fit is about cultivating more emotional intelligence and resilience.

Like strength, flexibility, and stamina are aspects of physical fitness; emotional intelligence, self-awareness, and stress resilience are aspects of emotional fitness.

Being emotionally fit means recognizing when we are becoming dysregulated and taking the necessary steps to bring ourselves back to a regulated state—without lashing out, blaming, wallowing in shame or self-loathing, or relying on self-harming coping strategies like overconsuming sugar or alcohol, watching mindless or negative programming, or whatever else you might do when you're feeling overwhelmed.

Emotional Fitness means having a regular practice of tuning heart and mind and body. It means getting to know yourself, feel your feelings, and developing a healthier relationship with your own emotions.

The Shift. Own your emotions; Own your life.

Emotional fitness is the ability to feel and express emotions in healthy ways without being overwhelmed or ruled by them. It's the ability to tell people we care about (and who care about us) when we are having a hard time and asking for support or a little more time to process before getting into that heated argument.

I believe the autoimmune issues I have dealt with much of my life are largely the result of learning to suppress and repress negative emotions. Perhaps the increasing prevalence of autoimmune disease, especially in women, is related to our increased suppression and repression of our emotions.

Like so many humans, I learned to survive with a combination of hiding my emotions and allowing them to pour out of me unchecked every now and again when I just couldn't contain them anymore. Instead of learning healthier ways of uncovering, examining, and processing my emotions, I allowed them to govern me. By focusing more and more on fantasies and false positivity, juxtaposed with extreme swings of negativity and self-loathing, I created more discordance in my body, which then, eventually manifested itself as dysfunction and disease.

I think a vast majority of humans have grown up with this default mode 'running the show'. If you grew up or spent time in an environment where it was not safe to be yourself, you likely learned coping strategies that might not serve you well in adulthood. Avoidance and anxiety about having feelings can create a cascade of emotions that leads to dysregulation.

Many of us live in a state of 'regular dysregulation.' Even if this is how it has been for most of your life and for most of the people around you, it does not have to be this way. This is really at the heart of this book. You can learn to

The Shift. Own your emotions; Own your life.

become more of a master of your own (positive and negative) emotions rather than letting them run your life.

Emotional Dysregulation:

Dysregulation, energetic turbulence, or internal incoherence, has become such a common state that many of us are wandering through our days and nights barely able to cope. It eats away at our energy and consumes huge portions of our lives.

The current epidemic rise in mass shootings, chronic illness, genocide, and suicide are symptoms of this underlying issue. Unfortunately, many of us use 'coping strategies' such as unhealthy eating, drugs and alcohol, and programming that hijacks our nervous system by controlling our emotions which make us less fit and more prone to emotional dysregulation.

Trying to handle the intensity of my emotions, and learning to deal with many people who have not learned how to feel or express emotions in healthy ways, has been a major theme in my life. I am passionate about shifting that in my own life and in the lives of others in all the ways I can.

It hurts us all when we are chronically dysregulated. Love is contagious. So is dysregulation and hate. By making emotional regulation a priority in your life, you can improve not only your own life, but you can also improve the lives of the people who are in your life, extending all the way to human societies and even entire ecosystems you belong to.

The Shift. Own your emotions; Own your life.

Intuition vs. Feelings:

For many of us, the ideas of feelings, emotions, and intuitive impulses are all mixed up. If you're like me, sometimes your feelings might feel like a tangled, messy ball of impossible intensity, with every thread containing another messy story and more tangled-up feelings.

I hope this book will help you learn to name and process your emotions more effectively, and take some of the mysterious and often chaotic sting out of them for you.

So, what's the difference between emotions, feelings, and intuitions?

In studying for this book, I quickly learned that there is no consensus about what any of these actually are. Different disciplines use different definitions, and many of us use emotions and feelings interchangeably.

Emotions are Constructed:

Meta studies done in the early 2000s revealed that the classical idea of 'universal emotions' does not hold up to cross-cultural scrutiny. The latest research suggests that our emotions are constructed, and the stories we tell ourselves about how we feel, in turn, influence how we process incoming data in the future.

Our brains are literally simulation machines, constructing our reality from a complex web of experiences and 'programming', especially from those earliest influences.

The Shift. Own your emotions; Own your life.

Feelings, Emotions, and Intuition:

We often use these terms interchangeably. In my quest to better understand and articulate what it means to be emotionally fit, I quickly ran into muddy waters. Various schools of study and thought agree and disagree. There is no consensus on a single definition for any of these terms.

Ultimately, many researchers have spent a lot of time and money concluding the same things any of us probably could: People have a lot of mixed feelings, and we are not very good at expressing them in healthy ways. We are both, seemingly ruled by our emotions, and also, mostly in agreement that too much emotion is bad and that overly emotional people are best avoided.

One problem arises in definitions. Many of us use 'feelings' and 'emotions' interchangeably, but it is worth making a distinction, at least for this book.

Keep in mind, these are working definitions meant to point toward concepts. All of these are complex. Feelings, emotions, and intuition are terms that humans have been exploring for as long as we have been keeping track of things.

I am not proposing that my definitions are the correct or only ones. I am setting these definitions here to ensure we have a common language, at least in the pages of this book. Let's not 'mistake the finger for the moon' and keep in mind this is simply my attempt to establish common ground to sow some seeds of healing and ultimately of living richer, more meaningful and fulfilling lives.

Emotions are the chemical and electromagnetic responses that our bodies (and microbiomes, and surrounding/connecting/entangled bodies) have all the time. They are constantly occurring and being processed, reacting and interacting with the chemistry and electromagnetic fields of everything else around us.

We are emotional beings, and emotions are essentially the neurochemical language of this 'meat machine' we call "my body".

Emotions really only get our conscious attention when our system perceives that something is amiss or needs us to shift our attention. Then we call them feelings.

Feelings are the stories we make up to explain what we notice, or how we are interpreting our emotions. They are often based on inaccurate, distorted, or incomplete interpretations of our emotions.

Feelings are not facts, but they are our interpretations of data or messages from our nervous system and sensory organs. Feelings contain important information but many of us do not take the time to learn the language of our emotions or reflect on what our feelings really mean.

We frequently blame other people and circumstances for our feelings and think that they are out of our control, but actually we have more control over both, our emotions and our feelings, than we like to think. Our thoughts create chemical cascades in our bodies, which in turn can create more, similar 'feelings'.

Intuition is that sensation of clarity we get when we are tuning in to our emotions with less of that misaligned discordance. I believe it comes from data that we are not consciously aware of but have access to. It is the sense we get when we become aware of a slight adjustment or shift in direction we can make to be in sync with our 'higher self', or the part of us that includes our consciousness,

The Shift. Own your emotions; Own your life.

subconsciousness, and what many call the superconsciousness (which I think of as our genetics, societal roles, place in history, etc).

I sometimes refer to this as alignment of our consciousness (what we are aware of) with our subconscious (memories and pheromones and hormones etc. that we are unaware of) and superconscious (the muti-generation and/or societal aspects—one could say our biology, sociology, and psychology). Intuitive impulses can also come from symbols and archetypical ideals.

Learning to listen to your own intuition is a skill worth investing time in, as it is one of the most valuable assets you have.

To me, intuition is a form of pattern recognition that my logical brain might not always be able to make linear sense of, but that my 'feeling' brain (often associated with the right hemisphere) knows.

To me, this is not supernatural. It is simply a natural skill most of us have not developed. Rather than thinking of it as 'mystical' or even metaphysical, intuition is a type of listening skill that can be developed. This type of 'knowing' can be thought of as the language of the right hemisphere of the brain, at least in some contexts.

Learning to listen to your own intuition is essentially learning your own language—the language of your own spirit or soul or psyche as well as your body (whether or not you consider these two separate things). It is how your greatest or highest-self communicates to you.

I have heard some describe intuition as the quiet, or small voice. I like to describe it as a 'whisper of clarity'.

The Shift. Own your emotions; Own your life.

By changing the stories we tell about our emotions, we can change how we feel. By changing how we feel, we can change the feedback loop. When we change the loop, we raise our energetic frequency and soothe the erratic eruptions and unconscious patterns playing out in our lives.

The feedback loop for changing our behaviors in order to help us change our stories is in our emotions, feelings, and intuition—it is all interconnected.

Let that sink in for a few minutes and circle back to it.

Asking the right questions is key to making the difference between success and failure in so much of life.

Feelings are often polarized. We think of them as "good" or "bad." They often result in, or are the result of, unbalanced thoughts.

We become aware of our feelings when they become more acute or when we consciously tap into our emotions. We can use our feelings and conscious thoughts as guidance to do the necessary work to transmute our weaknesses into strengths.

Your emotions, and the feelings that result from them, are telling you where you are balanced and unbalanced; where you are in and out of alignment. They are your body's signaling system, alerting you that something needs your attention.

At a foundational level, our animal bodies are programmed to seek prey, food, and reproductive opportunities and avoid discomfort, predators, and things that might harm us. Your brain is the control center for much of this, and your thoughts, or internal dialogue, play a significant role in

The Shift. Own your emotions; Own your life.

determining your internal chemistry, which in turn, impacts your perceptions of the world around and inside you.

According to some fascinating research by Brene Brown and her colleagues, there are more than 80 distinct feelings in the English language, but the average Westerner identifies most with only three: happy, sad, and mad.

When we learn to articulate our emotions or feelings with more nuance, it helps us process them and can lead to healthier relationships with ourselves and each other.

It is worth taking a look at the emotions wheel created by psychologist Dr. Robert Plutchik in the 1980s. Since its creation, it has been expanded and is a valuable resource for finding more words to describe your many nuanced feelings.

On some level, we can also 'boil them all down' to a binary perspective. From my perspective, all emotions can be reduced to essentially love and fear—expansion or moving towards something, and contraction, or recoiling away from something. If I step back far enough, I see that even fear is simply an 'underinformed or distorted expression of love on some level.'

Very often, we cover our fears with anger. Have you ever been in an argument with a child or a parent and felt they were angry to a degree that did not make sense to you? If so, perhaps you recognized at some point that really it was that they were actually afraid and that they were covering that fear, trying to cope with that feeling of existential threat with an outpouring of anger.

INVITATION TO ACTION: I invite you to pause and think about the last time you got angry with someone. This can be someone you care about or even a complete stranger or a public figure.

Before you get too revved up in remembering that anger, try to uncover what fear or insecurity is under that anger. Were you afraid of losing your freedom or autonomy? Where you afraid someone was going to get hurt or angry because someone did get hurt? Were you feeling insecure, unsafe, or uncertain?

Now, consider what is under that fear or insecurity. It is nearly always a deep love of something that leads us to become fearful of losing it or having it taken from us that leads us to become angry. This is why I say that under anger is always fear, and fear is simply underinformed, underdeveloped, or unconscious love.

Maybe it's as simple as loving life, and feeling that threatened somehow. Then chemical signals we get when we feel rejected or disrespected can feel like an existential threat if they are left unchecked, which is why becoming more self aware and learning to self-regulate is such an important life-skill for all of us, perhaps now more than ever.

This system of emotions driven by neurochemical and electromagnetic interactions is a necessary and beautifully designed aspect of life as we currently know it. It has been honed over many thousands or even millions of years. The vast majority of our chemical changes go unnoticed by our conscious minds.

The Shift. Own your emotions; Own your life.

When we become aware of an emotion, the story we tell ourselves about it becomes a feeling; we give it a name, and if we stop there, we integrate that into our reality as "I feel angry" or "I am feeling excited." This is fine and natural, but not likely to get us to the place where this is useful. Instead of stopping at that story, we can get curious and explore what we are truly desiring, and what of our own beliefs and values we are out of congruence with.

So next time you notice yourself telling a story about what you are feeling, try digging a bit deeper. See if you can give it a more specific name. See if you can find out what is underneath it. Bring it into the light and watch it dissolve and dissipate.

"It's a-half-past four and I'm shifting gear" Radar Love, by Golden Earring

Quantum Leaps & Shifts

A quantum leap is defined in the Merriam-Webster dictionary as: *An abrupt change, sudden increase, or dramatic advance.*

NOTE: Quantum leap {or shift} is rarely used in scientific contexts, but it originated as a synonym of quantum jump, which describes an abrupt transition (as of an electron, an atom, or a molecule) from one discrete energy state to another.

I find this helpful to think about when considering how to make significant changes in my own life. A quantum leap or shift is an abrupt change or a dramatic advance. It sometimes defies the 'logic' of everyday life, where we generally follow similar patterns and take small steps. Atomic habits and quantum leaps are interrelated, and they are both happening all the time.

Learning to harness the capacity of both these natural phenomena is part of what I am calling The Shift. Add a dash of 'improbability drive' from *The Hitchhiker's Guide to the Galaxy*, and now you have a method for dramatically up-leveling your life. You can change things quickly, and you can also make incremental, steady changes. It is not an 'either-or' situation. Rather, it is a 'both-and' aspect of this life.

By combining the practice of making consistent, small changes in your life with the practice of making abrupt changes and dramatic 'leaps' in your energetic state, you can create a life that is barely recognizable to your former self. It does require a combination of embracing the unknown — the Great Mystery of Life — while also building trust with yourself through consistent positive action. It also requires letting go of your limiting beliefs and shitty stories about yourself and creating a new sense of identity.

Sometimes a quantum shift might look like a dramatic change in location or physical circumstances, but always it is also a dramatic internal shift. You really can't have one without the other eventually.

I encourage you to consider that you can make meditation or focusing on shifting your energetic state a regular practice. In fact, if you prioritize this habit consistently, you can make much greater strides in creating a life that brings you more joy and satisfaction, more fulfillment, more love, more creativity — more of whatever you decide is most important for you in your life.

However, if you don't drop the old shit-story you keep telling about yourself, you are going to keep finding yourself back in the same old patterns of self-defeat.

Ask me how I know.

This probably sounds easier said than done. It is actually as easy to do it as it is to say it. Just do it. I mean, it might be hard, and you are very likely going to fail a lot of times, but doing will create the changes you desire.

Saying you want to do it can sometimes create the opposite result, especially if you say it while focusing on the feeling like you are not doing it. Ruminating on how you want things to be different can decrease your energetic state and spiral you into 'the pit of despair' or a low energetic state where you embody the victim-perpetrator-martyr mentality loop. Around and around you will go, feeling like you are stuck in *Groundhog Day*.

If you take your consistent actions from a low energetic state, you may cultivate a life that 'fits in' better with mainstream humanity, but it will remain unsatisfying and full of struggle.

If you can learn to raise your vibrational frequency first, get in touch with who you REALLY are, and who you REALLY want to be, and get into a higher energetic state, and THEN take consistent and inspired action, you might be amazed at the life you can create.

The Shift. Own your emotions; Own your life.

Emotional Hygiene is the term I will use in this book to refer to the process of transforming your sense of overwhelm and strong emotions into fuel for positive evolution in your life. Another way of thinking about it is good stress management. It's developing regular routines and habits that support your emotional fitness, so you can enjoy a more dynamic and satisfying, healthier and happier life.

When we examine our feelings, learn to ask better questions about them, and make processing and rebalancing them a regular part of our daily routine—along with so many other aspects of personal hygiene—we can begin to build the unique and beautifully rich lives we are capable of.

Much like brushing and flossing your teeth regularly can help keep them healthier, developing a regular practice of exploring your own emotions while taking full responsibility for them will improve the quality of your life magnificently.

Journaling is an excellent tool for self-inquiry and discovery. A regular journaling practice will help you develop better emotional hygiene. There are many variations of journaling, but I like to use a basic framework that includes some venting or releasing resentments, some organizing my obligations and prioritizing them, some dreaming or analyzing dreams, and some documenting or charting progress and failures. Doodles, colors, stickers, and specific types of journals (such as my gratitude journal or my releasing resentments journal) are all helpful for practicing good emotional hygiene.

I think of self-inquiry as a tool similar to dental floss or mouthwash. When used regularly, asking yourself good questions and answering yourself honestly is an important part of an effective emotional hygiene routine.

The Shift. Own your emotions; Own your life.

I have gathered questions used by many wise philosophers who have come before me (Alan Watts, Victor Frankl, Byron Katie, Carl Jung, James Hollis, Brené Brown, and John Demartini just to name a few) to create a framework that I find most helpful in cleaning up messy emotional states.

By asking yourself these questions when you notice you are feeling dysregulated or overwhelmed by emotion, you can learn to use the energy that would be squandered on strong emotional outbursts. You can stop reacting to life and start becoming the master of your own destiny. You can learn to take responsibility and control your own emotional states.

As long as we are blaming any outside forces for our internal state, we will be stuck in a reactive state, blown around by the winds of our emotions and by the emotions of others.

This is the key that nearly all successful people have figured out, and you can figure it out too. It does not require any special equipment or anyone else to help you. Anyone who can ask and answer questions can benefit from this process.

You can gain more positive momentum in life by learning to 'smooth out' the extreme emotional reactions in your life. You can learn to catch them sooner. Practice recognizing them as potential fuel to propel you forward, rather than allowing them to knock you off course all the time.

When you realize you are feeling overwhelmed and narrating a self-defeating story or thinking the same bad-feeling thought over and over again, stop and ask yourself these simple questions. If you can, sit down with a pen and

The Shift. Own your emotions; Own your life.

paper, at a keyboard, or record yourself asking and
answering so you can revisit your answers.

Coherence

Did you know your heart actually sends more information to
your brain than your brain sends to your heart? Heart-brain
coherence is a relatively new field of study that show when
our hearts and brains are out of sync it's like we are
disconnected from ourselves. Studies show that simply
slowing down our breathing and focusing on our heart and
positive feelings such as gratitude can increase our heart-
brain coherence.

The vagus nerve is the longest nerve in the body and it
connects all our major body systems, including our heart
and brain. Vagal toning has also been shown to be an
effective way to improve our overall coherence. More
coherence means more capacity to do the things you want,
and to bring other people into your frequency and co-
regulate with you.

INVITATION TO ACTION: The next time you
catch your brain looping around a dysregulated or reactive
thought, make a mental note of it and if you can, write
down the exact thought, or record a short voice-note or
video of it. Then, make some time to see if you can
untangle or dig a bit deeper underneath that thought and

discover something new or uncover something you have hidden from yourself.

Start by writing down the thought. You might choose to frame it with a distancing phrase such as "The story I am telling myself in my head right now is [fill in with the thought or disempowering story].

Then, be courageous and compassionate, and get curious.

A good first set of questions to ask is:

Is that really true?

Is that the whole truth and nothing but the truth?

How would I feel if it wasn't true, or if I didn't believe it was true?

How is it serving me to think this is true?

What aspect of me is telling this story?

Can I find a better-feeling thought?

Are there other perspectives I can tell the story from that feel less disempowering?

How might this be the best thing that ever happened to me?

If your thoughts are blaming someone else, you can ask:

Where do I do this too?

How is it serving me to blame or shame this person?

The Shift. Own your emotions; Own your life.

What do I really want from this interaction or relationship?

What is a more positive and productive thought?

You might be tempted to think, "It isn't serving me at all," and shame yourself for having the thought. Or you might think, "It is serving me by helping me set healthier boundaries."

I encourage you to go a bit deeper and circle back through the questions at least a few times. See if you can loosen the stranglehold on your thoughts just a little bit. Keep in mind, the objective is not to get to some 'right answer', rather, the whole point is to start to train your brain to not be so rigid, and to create possibility where before there was none.

Put a little bit more space into it, even if you need to use a trick at first, like counting or a deep inhale and exhale. If you must distract yourself, see if you can choose a healthier distraction or a less destructive one.

If you are beating yourself up internally, try saying the thought out loud and see how it sounds, but do be mindful that the intention of this exercise is not to be self-abusive or shame yourself in any way.

The intention is to get curious. Give it a genuine inquiry. Would you say that to a child or elder who you love?

Remember that those parts of you that are most unruly and illogical are like your internal child self or perhaps your untamed and wounded rebellious teen self. I invite you to see if you can be more compassionate towards yourself. Pretend you are someone you love and give yourself a little more grace.

Suppression vs. Processing

In order to process our feelings in healthy ways, we need to allow ourselves to feel them. Emotional intelligence—or the ability to perceive, interpret, demonstrate, control, evaluate, and use emotions to communicate with and relate to others effectively and constructively—is a major key to living a healthy and happy life.

Like other types or aspects of intelligence, most of us come with various amounts of emotional intelligence. Luckily, we can also cultivate and develop more of it with practice. When we cultivate more emotional intelligence and learn to use what we have naturally more effectively, we can get better at identifying and processing our feelings, and also the feelings and emotions of those around us.

In our modern society, suppressing or repressing our feelings seems to be a more common response than feeling and processing them. This is more understandable when you realize that most of us do not know how to handle intense feelings, even positive ones, without spiraling into dysregulation.

When compared to dysregulation, suppression and repression are more logical choices, but they are still not our healthiest, or best options over the long run.

Repression is essentially unconscious suppression. It is the outcome of a great number of our modern pastimes, such as escaping into entertainment or overconsumption, and also the age-old practice of telling ourselves self-defeating stories that aren't even true.

75

The Shift. Own your emotions; Own your life.

When we choose to distract ourselves and overconsume food, mind-numbing media, or alcohol and other drugs to escape our own feelings, we are generally repressing them. Sometimes we do this more consciously and suppress them by choice. In any case, this is just not healthy in the long run.

It's like having dozens of apps open on your phone all the time in the background. They might not be doing a lot, but each unprocessed emotion is taking up bandwidth. Sooner or later, with too much unprocessed 'gunk', systems start to malfunction, overheat, and just do not work right.

Usually our bodies try to warn us that something is up with feelings like 'something is amiss', a new pain, a rash, a mood, poor digestion, or that pervasive sense of general anxiety so many of us live with for long periods of time.

Over time, when we do not listen to what our bodies are trying to tell us, and we do not check in with and address the stories our brains are feeding us, it leads to chronic stress, incoherence, and increasing dysregulation.

Many of us turn to sensory numbing coping strategies to distract ourselves from the increasing sense of anxiety and disease that comes from living in this chronically repressed state.

It sucks away our vibrance and our potential. We become less capable and less present. We enjoy the richness and possibilities of our lives less and less.

Suppressing and repressing our emotions is what we do when we push them aside, tell ourselves they are not appropriate, or believe we are not allowed to feel them. Suppression and repression is not the same as processing.

The Shift. Own your emotions; Own your life.

There is a tendency in our modern world to shun anyone who shows too much emotion. Meanwhile, people who lose the ability to feel emotions often lose their ability to make meaning of their lives and find it difficult to want to survive.

Women are generally criticized for being overly sensitive and men are generally criticized for being insensitive. Of course, these are generalizations, but they are generally true. I hope I can show you how we can all benefit from learning to feel and process our emotions in healthier ways.

Having strong feelings does not have to mean being emotionally dysregulated or out of control. It can mean feeling more deeply and enjoying a more meaningful life without being overwhelmed.

Emotional fitness can include becoming more aware of and more responsible for your own emotions. It can mean living a rich, more fulfilling, dynamic life full of meaning and purpose.

On the surface, it might seem that those who are the most successful are not as emotional as those who seem frequently overwhelmed by emotions.

While this is partially true, those who truly enjoy their lives have learned to feel their feelings and respond to them in healthier ways. It is those who learn to listen to their emotions, feel and process them in productive and healthy ways who find the deepest meaning in life. They feel plenty.

The key difference is learning to process them in healthy ways. Suppression and repression of our feelings simply stores that energy in the body and psyche, where it can become stagnant, distorted, and unhealthy.

The Shift. Own your emotions; Own your life.

Suppressed emotions often spill over and out at inopportune times and sometimes in shocking ways. Ultimately, this taxes and stresses our bodies' systems and can become excess weight, clutter, disorder, dysfunction, and disease. It can also ruin relationships which can suck the sense of success and joy from our lives over time.

Acute and Chronic Dysregulation

I want to point out an important distinction between acute and chronic dysregulation. Acute dysregulation is a natural, healthy response to being alive.

There will be things that happen that knock you off your feet, literally and metaphorically. To wish for no dysregulation, no suffering, no problems, is the wish of a dead person. That is not how life works. Birth and death are often violent, and many details in between can be bewildering.

Chronic dysregulation is what happens when we let our negative and self-defeating thoughts 'run amuck' and rule our lives. A repeating thought, left unchecked, can become a mood, and a mood, left unchanged, can become a personality trait and eventually, a part of us we call our identity. This is why regular self-reflection and attitude adjustment are such important keys.

Your brain's job is to keep you safe and alive. It is natural for it to point out what is wrong, look for problems, and even obsess over things you can't change. But you are not your brain.

Your brain is a part of you, and often a very child-like part at that. One of your brain's main functions is to keep you safe and maintain homeostasis. This means you will naturally notice things that seem alarming all the time, even if they are really not. Most of the thoughts your brain comes up with are not really true, especially if you have not spent much time consciously cultivating discernment.

One of the most important things you can learn to do is to train your brain to serve you and your goals, rather than

79

allowing your brain and the thoughts it comes up with to steer your life unchecked.

There will be days you feel great, and other days you feel downright crummy. Many things will happen around you that you won't be able to control. You will sometimes get blindsided by things in life, no matter how well-prepared, resilient, and fit you are. This is natural and normal and part of a healthy system your body has developed to help alert you to dangers and possibilities.

Acute dysregulation is normal and may be unavoidable to an extent. However, there is much you can do to become more adept at feeling your emotions without becoming dysregulated and to lessen the time you remain in a dysregulated state.

Chronic dysregulation is avoidable and also can be turned around and even healed. Chronic dysregulation left unchecked, leads to chronic illness.

Learning to become more emotionally fit is not about never becoming dysregulated. It is about learning to recognize when you are dysregulated and bringing yourself back to a regulated state more rapidly. I liken it to recognizing when my guitar is out of tune and taking a minute to tune it back up before playing the next song.

If you let every unexpected 'disaster' or crisis be a valid reason to veer off course, then you will go through life reacting to the outside world, a slave to circumstance rather than the master of your own destiny. You are likely to wind up like the vast majority of people—never experiencing the life they dream of, or perhaps not even dreaming at all. That would be a tragedy.

The Shift. Own your emotions; Own your life.

Instead, you can learn to examine your emotions, dive into them from a healthy perspective, and see what they are telling you about your life. Use them as information, be grateful for them, and learn to bring yourself back to a centered state more quickly so that you don't get knocked off course so often or for so long.

You can shift from living in hindsight to living in foresight; from reacting to responding. It simply takes doing it. It gets easier with practice.

You can learn to recognize the signs that you are dysregulated more quickly so you can take steps to bring yourself back into a more coherent and calm state.

You can cultivate healthy skills and strategies that help you grow from your challenges rather than feel beaten down by failure over time.

You can expand your capacity to feel your emotions in greater detail, gleaning more of the valuable information your body is trying to communicate to you, without feeling victimized by your own system. This is the key to developing healthy human relationships that don't end in devastation and drama.

Let's go back to the analogy of tuning my guitar. When I play it a lot, don't play for a long time, play in fluctuating weather, travel, or play particular songs that are high energy, it goes out of tune. That is not a failure or a problem. It is natural.

Being out of tune doesn't mean my guitar is defective or broken or useless. It simply means that I must make tuning it up a regular part of playing. There is a skill to it, and it gets easier with practice.

The Shift. Own your emotions; Own your life.

Anytime I am about to play my guitar, I tune it up first. If I'm playing more than a short set, I'll tune it up periodically as needed or when I get an opportunity to give it a quick check.

This is a good analogy for how we can think of emotional fitness and self-mastery. The objective is not to never get 'out of tune.' In fact, the more vibrantly we live our lives, the harder we play, the more frequently we are likely to need to tune things up.

The goal is to develop the skills and awareness needed to keep ourselves tuned up to the best of our ability so we can be the best we can be and enjoy playing over the long run.

You may have heard the saying, "Every person lives two lives, and the second one begins when they realize they only have one." Similarly, I think that every person makes The Shift when they realize there is not just One Big Shift. Rather, The Shift is that subtle but important decision to be responsible for your own thoughts, feelings, and actions, a decision we all get to make again and again.

The Shift happens when you begin to cheerfully accept and appreciate the potential and opportunities that every challenge in life presents to you and do your best to do your best. It's about being ready to be ready; being willing to succeed at failing. It's about being confident, courageous, and always aiming to improve, with great humility.

Neurochemistry Basics: The Science of Emotion in Motion

Science has made great strides in helping us understand what influences our emotional states, and it's always still learning. Your brain is always mixing up different chemical cocktails which in turn effect your perceptions and predictions.

Here are a few of the core neurochemicals that we know play a major role in how we feel, act, and respond. These chemicals impact our motivation, mood, regulation, and resilience. They are not the only 'players' but they are the ones we know the most about.

We won't get deep into these here, but having a basic understanding of these molecules can help you work with your natural biology rather than against your brain and body.

Here are five key neurochemicals that influence our emotions and how we can use awareness of them in practical, powerful ways.

Dopamine: The Motivation Molecule

Dopamine drives desire, anticipation, reward-seeking, and habit formation. When it's balanced you feel motivated, curious, and energized to take action. When dopamine is out of sync you may procrastinate, feel unmotivated, or seek quick hits (scrolling, snacking, etc.) instead of meaningful progress.

You can support balanced dopamine by breaking big tasks into small wins, celebrating completion, and adding novelty and visual cues for success in your external environment

83

The Shift. Own your emotions; Own your life.

(think inspiring art, t-shirts, motivational posters, organized closet, clean kitchen…).

Norepinephrine: The Focus Amplifier

Norepinephrine drives alertness, attention, and your readiness for challenge. When norepinephrine is balanced you feel alert, focused, and capable of tackling your to-do list. When this molecule is out of sync you might feel scattered, wired, or foggy and unable to start.

You can support healthy norepinephrine balance by moving your body, splashing cold water on your face, or using a timer to create urgency with a short timer.

Cortisol: The Stress Regulator

Cortisol drives your body's stress response and energy availability. When it's balanced you feel resilient, and able to navigate pressure without collapsing. When cortisol is out of balance, you may become tense, reactive, and overwhelmed, or swing into shutdown.

You can support healthy cortisol levels by learning to breathe deeply. Pause. Reframe your thinking. Get grounded in the present moment. Learn to let go of stress or use it as a cue to relax rather than spiraling deeper into it.

Oxytocin: The Connection Chemical

Oxytocin drives our trust, bonding, and sense of emotional safety. When oxytocin is in healthy balance, you feel safe, connected, open to others and to your own heart. When cortisol is out of sync you may want to isolate, numb out, or struggle to ask for support--even when you need it most.

The Shift. Own your emotions; Own your life.

You can support healthy oxytocin levels by connecting with someone you trust or petting an animal. Offering kind words and even hugging yourself can help give you an oxytocin boost. Humming, singing, or chanting can also increase your oxytocin.

Endorphins: The Natural Pain Relievers

Endorphins drive euphoria, resilience, and relief from emotional or physical pain. When endorphins are well-balanced you feel uplifted and capable of riding life's waves with lightness. When endorphins are out of balance, you may feel dull, flat, and joyless--or chase high-stimulation just to feel something.

You can cultivate healthy endorphins in your own body. When you laugh, dance, sing, or stretch you are releasing endorphins and changing your experience. Even a little can go a long way.

Understanding these chemicals gives you a deeper layer of emotional literacy. They don't replace your feelings—they help explain why certain tools work better in certain moments. They're not the whole picture, but they are *part* of how you shift.

Later, we'll return to this and give you more ways to work with your chemistry, especially when you feel stuck in self-sabotage or struggling to reboot. For now, just remember:

You're not broken—you're bioelectric. And that means you can be rewired, not just through willpower, but through small, smart shifts in behavior and awareness.

The Shift. Own your emotions; Own your life.

INVITATION TO ACTION: Think about the last week. Can you identify times in the last week when a neurochemical imbalance was driving behavior that did not seem to make sense? Looking at your behaviors through the lens of neurochemistry, can you think of healthier ways that you might rebalance a specific molecule, such as oxytocin, cortisol, or norepinephrine?

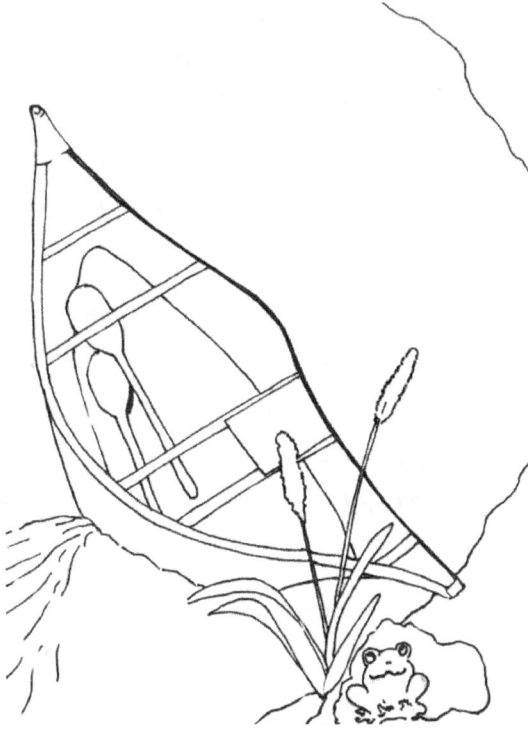

The Parable of the Empty Boat

A young monk who was studying to master inner peace was trying to meditate but he kept being distracted by the noise and dramas of the people around him. The dogs barking and chickens clucking, and children shrieking were a constant annoyance.

Eventually, to find peace and quiet, he hiked up a nearby mountain and took his boat onto a tranquil lake to get more peace and quiet to continue his practice.

87

The Shift. Own your emotions; Own your life.

He put his boat into the water and paddled out to the center of the lake. He sat in the boat and smiled, exhaling a deep sigh of relief, appreciating that he was finally free from the distractions that had been keeping him from finding the deep sense of peace he was after.

As he floated on the calm waters, he closed his eyes, breathed deeply, and allowed the serenity of the surroundings to wash over him.

Just as he was beginning to feel the first stirrings of deep inner peace, he heard the sound of another boat approaching.

Annoyed by the disturbance, he opened his eyes and saw a boat heading straight toward him. Irritated, he shouted at the boatman to steer away.

"Why can't I get any deep inner peace and quiet, even when I remove myself from all the distractions of the city?" he lamented in frustration.

"Turn away, you fool!" He exclaimed angrily.

"You are paddling straight towards me and I am the only other boat on this lake!"

He was overcome with rage and stood up in his boat and shouted even louder. "You there! Steer away!"

He felt himself getting hot and feeling incredulous that whoever was in the other boat would be so inconsiderate and careless.

But as the boat drew closer, he noticed it was empty, simply drifting with the current, the same as his boat was.

The Shift. Own your emotions; Own your life.

There was no one at the helm, no one to blame.

In that moment, the monk's anger dissolved, and he laughed heartily as he realized the futility of his reaction.

He understood that the anger and frustration he felt at this and so many other distractions were of his own making. The distraction and irritation were all in his own mind.

Both the boats drifted there naturally because of the current under the surface of the water in the lake.

So often, the sources of our frustrations are not intentional aggressions or personal attacks, but simply the inevitable flow of life, just like in this story.

It does no good to try to control the outside world to avoid disturbances. Instead, we can learn to calm ourselves from the inside, navigate our lives with a steady mind, and master our own reactions.

There will always be things that come up and have the potential to 'rock our boat' in this life. The key is to learn to keep ourselves steady and calm so that fewer and fewer things disrupt our sense of well-being.

If we let every disruption, every turbulence, be a reason to allow ourselves to get knocked off course, or into a dysregulated state, then we are likely to have a miserable time getting nowhere.

CHAPTER 3

NO ONE IS COMING

You are the secret sauce you've been waiting for...

We are all familiar with the saying, "With great power comes great responsibility," but have you considered that the inverse is also true?

"With great responsibility comes great power."

Responsibility literally means being able to respond. The first step in making a positive change in your life is to realize that no one else can make that change for you. No one else will care more about your life or put more time, effort, or attention into achieving your desires than you.

Let that sink in because it's at the heart of the shift you're going to make. Once you recognize that you are not living the life you desire--and that this is due to the choices you are or aren't making, the actions you are and are not taking, as well as the energetic framework from which you are making them--then you are ready to take responsibility for living your one, true, amazingly fantastic life.

Please note, I am NOT saying you don't deserve help or that you should not ever ask for and receive help. It's just that the help you receive from others will be immeasurably more effective, and actually helpful, if you first help yourself.

If you just throw up your hands and wait for others to help you, you may get some help, but it will not last long if you don't eventually take the helm of your own life and learn to help yourself, at least most of the time.

I am also not saying that you deserve all the unfortunate or terrible things that have happened to you, or that anyone can control all the external or internal factors in their lives. I AM saying that you CAN control more of your life than you might think, simply by learning to control the way you respond to your own emotions and feelings.

You must decide to take full responsibility for your own life in order to live it fully. And as far as I know, you are the only one in all of existence currently qualified to do so.

The good news is that once you decide to step fully into becoming your vibrantly alive, creative self, you will find yourself opening doors you might never have dreamed of. In time, you might even find yourself able to 'draw new doors' and achieve dreams as regularly as you can bring them fully into your consciousness.

Does this mean you will never suffer or struggle again? No.

Does it mean you won't feel the grief that comes from losing what you love sometimes? Sigh. Unfortunately not. No.

The Shift. Own your emotions; Own your life.

Does it mean you won't ever feel the guilt or shame that comes from making choices that are not aligned with your truest, most authentic self again? Probably not.

I seriously doubt it.

Human experience is full of dualities and contrasts. I believe that you really can't get it wrong, and it never ends—at least, it lasts this entire lifetime. I don't know what happens after that, so I won't pretend that I do.

This might seem anticlimactic, but it's also where it gets exciting! While this realization may feel overwhelming, it's the very key to unlocking your full power.

Many people never dare to take the reins of their own lives and play a conscious role in cultivating their life experiences. Congratulate yourself, and 'buckle up,' because some of this could be a bumpy ride.

Probably the most important key to making the most of your life is taking personal responsibility for it.

Whatever upbringing you did or didn't get, whatever stories you have built your identity around, ultimately, you are the one who will live with every decision you make. It's worth taking a regular pause to reflect on your decisions and making sure they align with your values.

Living out of alignment with our personal values is the cause of a great deal of dysregulation among us.

An important part of this is realizing that you are more capable than you might think. Maybe you've been led to believe that you are broken, defective, or dysfunctional. I assure you, brave one, there is no single label that can fully describe you. Your untapped potential is far greater than that.

Right now, you might be thinking, "Yeah, but…" or "Not me, because…" or "You don't know…"

The thing is, as I have mentioned several times already, I have seen and experienced a lot of those parts that most people hide and don't want anyone to see. I have seen the dark threads and shadowy sides of highly esteemed families and shared the bright hopes that run in the gutters and dark alleys; so many unseen by most of humanity.

I assure you; you are no more and no less worthy of love than any other creature on this earth, and certainly no more or less valuable than any other human.

Consider the thousands of humans who have triumphed against greater odds than this. Consider the starlings, ravens, coyotes, the monarch butterflies, the leatherback turtles, and the whale sharks. Consider the unique resilience of a gnarled bristlecone pine tree growing in the cracks of stone cliffs for five thousand years against the freezing dry wind. You and I and they are all part of this grand thing we call life.

You are stronger, wiser, and more capable than you think. Life is resilient and incredible, and you are a part of it. So, snuggle in tight, and let's begin. Again.

No one is coming to save you.

I will repeat it because I know this is hard to accept sometimes.

No one is coming.

There is no knight in shining armor, no fairy godmother, no genie in a bottle, no baby Jesus, no twin flame lover coming to save the day.

Even if there were, no one else could 'make you' into the person you want to become.

You are the only one qualified to take up the full-time occupation of becoming your best self. Everyone else is already busy, being themselves. So who you become is at least in large part, entirely up to you.

Yes, there are aspects of you that are pre-baked in. You might say the hand you are dealt is your fate, and how you play it is your destiny. I like the analogy of the warp and the weft in weaving.

Some of the threads of our life are indeed, predetermined, or at least, they seem to be. Other parts, however--those are the conscious choices we make and also the unconscious habits and patterns we undertake.

Those are the parts that are entirely up to you, whether you want to take conscious responsibility for them or not.

The good news is you can start today! You can stop waiting for someone or something else to come along and save you, make things better, or help you figure out how to clean up your mess. Everyone else is busy with their own lives, so any time they have left over for you will be just that--leftovers.

You are worth much more than crumbs and scraps. You are worthy of your own whole, unconditional love.

The Shift. Own your emotions; Own your life.

You are enough. You have always been enough. You will always be enough. Also, you can be more, or less.

Change is our only constant. No one else will ever care more about your life than you do.

Why not give it your best shot?

What is the alternative?

Are you really going to settle for mediocrity when you could give yourself your very best effort, even if your odds of absolute success are slim? As they say, you miss 100% of the shots you don't take.

I am sure you have heard all this before. I hope I can convince you to take positive action today. You don't need permission. You don't have to wait for any special revelation. You can begin today, right now, with a simple internal shift.

What is one thing you can do today that your future self will thank you for tomorrow?

Take a moment and contemplate this. Not simply in the broad sense of changing your mindset, although this is great, but in a practical sense. You could do the dishes, put your laundry away, clean out a shelf in the closet, or sweep the porch. You could paint or draw or complete a Spanish lesson. You could drink more water, go for a walk, have a salad, or not eat that cookie. You could do ten pushups or five minutes of deep breathing.

You get the idea. There are probably infinite options.

I encourage you to contemplate this question, but not too long, and then take some action. Right now. Do the thing.

The Shift. Own your emotions; Own your life.

Do SOMEthing. A thing. Start where you are and do the best you can with what you have.

➡ **INVITATION TO ACTION:** I invite you to pause for a few minutes, take out a piece of paper, start a video, or a note for yourself and write down or read this question out loud to yourself:

What is one thing I can do today that my future self will thank me for tomorrow?

I challenge you to come up with five to ten answers then choose ONE and do it. Right now.

You could set a timer for 2 or 3 minutes and brainstorm answers that way or set a minimum bar of at least ten and keep going until you have filled that quota or time allotment. Not all the answers will be great, most likely. The point is to invite your own brain to connect the dots between right now and tomorrow and find some simple way of improving your life, and actually DO it.

The point is not to come up with fantastic answers, though you might surprise yourself and come up with some good ones. The point is to practice improving your life, to increase your level of self-trust, and to begin the habit of taking swift action. So get to it. I will wait.

By the way, setting a timer is an easy way to encourage your more creative side to come out and play. It can be a very helpful tool, especially for brainstorming and for finishing short tasks.

Did you do the thing?

The Shift. Own your emotions; Own your life.

Great! You Rock!

If not, please, just pause briefly and do it. If so, great! You are off to a good start on this self-mastery journey.

You can raise your own consciousness. It does take practice to build momentum, and it does get easier over time. Even as it does, life will continue to unfold in ways that surprise and sometimes delight you. No one gets out alive, and the challenges of becoming your best self are ongoing.

Really though, go do the thing. You will feel a tiny bit better. I promise.

You don't have to become anything, and you don't owe anyone anything. However, you probably have a lot of untapped potential that you can still grow into, and you might want to.

You are the only one of your particular kind, the only one exactly like you in this exact position in space and time. You owe it to yourself to find out more about what you can do, don't you?

Believe me, I do know it's hard sometimes. Our brains naturally look for and find whatever is missing, wrong, or potentially dangerous. It is your brain's job to try to keep you alive, so it is always on the lookout for what is potentially dangerous, what is different, and what seems out of place.

This is one of the main reasons why getting started with a big change is so hard. Your brain is likely to resist any change at first, no matter how much you know it is the best thing for you.

The Shift. Own your emotions; Own your life.

Even if everything is fine, an undisciplined or dysregulated mind will spiral into the 'pit of despair' again and again. Trauma loops and self-defeating behaviors devour entire lifetimes. Let's not let that be you or your story.

With great responsibility comes great power.

Perfection is the enemy of progress.

You got this.

Recognize, Realize, and Decide to take responsibility for your life.

So, you've realized you are unhappy and something needs to change… This is great!

Now what?

When you recognize that you are unhappy or in a state of self-induced suffering, take note of all the signs.

Don't beat yourself up! This is a good thing!

To make The Shift, it's essential to acknowledge your dissatisfaction with the way things currently are. The question then becomes:

What will you do about it?

What to do now? Mope around, pout, and miss out? Get what you get and like it? Blame someone else? Play the *'look what you made me do'* game and make things even worse?

How about this? Take the reins, the wheel, the helm of your life story, and dare to be the responsible adult in your own life.

You are the main character, the most impressive villain, and the absolute hero of your life story.

Even if you refuse to own this aspect of yourself, you have still made a choice. No one else can live your life. Some people will disapprove, no matter what you do.

What matters most is that YOU approve of what you do, and when you realize you don't…

The Shift. Own your emotions; Own your life.

You can continue to wallow and whine, spin your wheels in the muck, thrash about madly… or you can learn to 'simmer down,' make The Shift, and take responsibility for yourself and your life.

Is it finally time? Are you ready?

Instead of telling yourself another story about whose fault it is—who did or didn't do something that caused you to not do or say the things you wanted—just stop telling that self-defeating story.

I know, I know, "but…this, that, and the other thing." Really though, just stop.

Shift your focus to what you do want. Recognize that your life is your responsibility. Everyone else is living their own lives. **This one is yours.**

It may seem counterintuitive, but you must make yourself your number one priority, even if, and especially if, you are caring for small children, parents, or others who depend on you. If you model to them that their needs take priority over yours, you could end up so battered, bitter, and bewildered that no one else seems to care for you the way you care for others.

Please, try not to use the people you love as an excuse for not blooming into your fullest capacity. They probably wouldn't want you to do that 'for them', any more than you would want them to do that 'for you'.

This is a mistake I see so many people make—and I've made it myself many times. We use our love or sense of duty to what is 'right' as a reason to sacrifice ourselves and not pursue our truest desires. In doing so, we squander so much of our lives.

The Shift. Own your emotions; Own your life.

We wind up feeling diminished, repressed, and sulky or bitter, rather than excited, vibrant, and exuberant to be alive. Then, we spend most of our precious energy trying to manipulate or coerce others into giving us back what we tried to give them.

The problem with this approach is that no one else asked you to make them and their life a priority over your own. If you try to leverage this to get them to reciprocate, they are likely to feel resentful and disconnected from you, rather than feeling all the gratitude you might think you deserve. If you are lucky, your children will eventually grow up to make their own lives their priority, not yours. You are on your own. You only owe yourself your self.

Even if you are resolved to prioritize the needs of someone else as your own, that does NOT mean that sacrificing your own wellbeing is necessary or even helpful. In fact, learning to care for your own needs is an essential part of being a caretaker.

Minding the Gap

"Between stimulus and response there is a space. In that space is our power to choose our response. In our response lies our growth and freedom." ~Viktor Frankl

We think the journey looks like this:

your dream life

you are here

But actually it looks more like this:

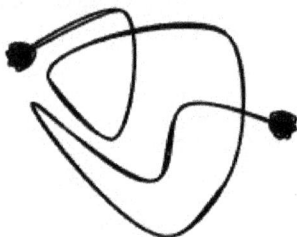

Mine looks more like this:

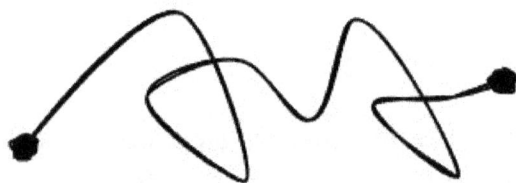

With more Emotional Fitness
it might be more like this:

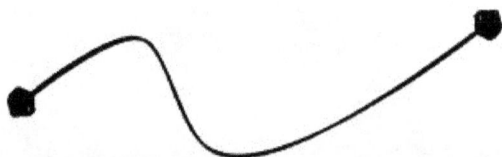

The Shift. Own your emotions; Own your life.

The distance between where we are and where we want to be is the cause of a great deal of self-inflicted suffering. It can also be the source of inspiration and motivation.

Often, we reach a point in our lives where we look around and feel dissatisfied with the life we have created. When we let too much time go by without checking in with ourselves or keeping up with maintenance and upgrades, the gap between what we think we will become and what we are grows.

Gaps might seem like a bad thing, but these gaps represent potential and spaces we can grow into. They often lead to what people used to call a 'midlife crisis'—the crisis of realizing that you are not living your life authentically, in accordance with who you want to be or who you really are. This seems to be a common aspect of the human condition.

This is natural. It happens to pretty much everyone in some way or another. Try not to beat yourself up about it—you don't need to. As it turns out, life will do plenty of that for you.

The gaps between who you are and who you want to be create a general sense of dis-ease or tension. Eventually this tension builds up, and the desire to ease the tension could end up propelling you forward or pulling your dreams and aspirations back a bit. One is not inherently better than the other, but it's helpful to regularly reflect on which option is the best one for you in your current stage of life.

The best remedy for the tension caused by this increasing gap is to regularly check in with your current state, and your expected or desired state, and actively work to bring them closer together. This usually involves being more practical and realistic with your expectations while also doing the work required to make progress toward the life you want to create.

This is where I urge you to push yourself forward into the gap and find out what you can do, more than reducing your dreams to make them more attainable. Cultivating a healthy relationship to the gaps in your life can be a super power, as much as having an unhealthy relationship to them can be like kryptonite.

If you regularly lament that you are not in great physical shape while eating ice cream and chips and looking at pictures of super-fit people, for example, you are increasing the gap. If you decide you are going to be happy being overweight, you could be decreasing the gap. Both of these are unhealthy, suboptimal strategies for dealing with the discomfort the gap causes in us.

Yes, I see you. In fact, I am you. That is how I know: when you increase the gap, you are likely to feel increasingly miserable as the distance between what you are and what you want to be continues to grow. If you use this as a reason to punish yourself or reward the wrong behaviors in yourself, it can really slow down your progress.

I have struggled with overeating and overconsuming various substances over many periods of my life. After I gave birth to my son, for example, instead of shedding the ample pregnancy weight I had gained, I continued to balloon until I was approaching 300 pounds. This is what can happen when we keep making the same poor choices again and again instead of shifting our direction.

It is not easy to turn around or shift direction when you have built up momentum going the wrong way, but it is worth it, and I know you can do it, because I have done it.

The Shift. Own your emotions; Own your life.

It wasn't easy, especially at first, but I decided to change my relationship with food and with my own body, and I did. Eventually, it got much easier, and now I have maintained a much healthier weight of about 150 pounds (plus or minus 10 pounds) for more than a decade.

Instead of increasing that gap, look at people you admire or things you want and take small steps to bring yourself closer to that.

At the very least, take your foot off the gas pedal and stop driving yourself in the wrong direction.

Go for a walk outside. Make regular time in your life to stretch, breathe, and let go of stress. Dance more.

Invest time in your relationships, including your relationship with your own body. Start a savings or investment account. Clean your room. Do the dishes. Get a massage. Say "no thanks" to that bag of chips. You will feel progressively better. It really can be that simple.

Life's challenges can manifest in various areas. Whether it's your body, your relationships, your finances, or your career that feels unsatisfactory, the first step is to notice and acknowledge that you are not happy with where you are. Then decide and begin to make the shift towards a more satisfying life.

It may not feel like it, especially at first, but realizing you are unhappy with your life really is a good thing, because it is you becoming aware that you want to make a change. That awareness can be the beginning of a more meaningful, satisfying, and beautiful existence.

The Shift. Own your emotions; Own your life.

Maybe you feel like you're not really stepping into your full potential. Maybe illness, death, or despair has sunk its hooks deeply into you and is threatening to take you down.

Life has no shortage of challenging details and situations. The trick is to learn to use them as inspirations to make things better, rather than using them as reasons to make things even harder.

Maybe you once dreamed of exotic travel and passionate weekends, but now life seems to be passing you by, and you are beginning to think it may be too late…

Perhaps, like me, you were sure you would be 'independently wealthy' and collecting seashells and polished glass on a beach every sunrise and sunset by now…

 Yet, somehow, some-- or maybe even most --of it hasn't quite panned out the way you hoped (yet).

Some of us refuse to pay attention to the signs until we reach a real crisis. Incarceration, disease, death, or sudden severe injury is often the catalyst that finally inspires us to make a significant shift in our lives. Realizing we are miserable or finding ourselves unable to tolerate the conditions we have created can be the wake-up call we finally heed.

Am I saying everything is your fault and should be under your control? No, I'm not saying that at all.

Am I saying you can control everything, even in yourself? Nope. Not at all.

I AM saying that you can learn to control yourself more consciously, more of the time, more successfully—and

The Shift. Own your emotions; Own your life.

by doing so, you CAN have more potential positive influence in the world. If nothing else, you'll live a more vibrant and satisfying life than if you don't.

Remember, an important aspect of minding the gap is to recognize that the gap is also that space of potential. It's perfectly fine to take your time as you navigate your personal journey towards your goals. As long as you are moving towards your goals (and your goals are moving you towards the person you want to be), or adjusting course when you recognize you are off-track, then you are likely to enjoy your journey more often than not.

"Failure is guaranteed; success is not." —Tom Bilyeu

Failure is a natural outcome if you want to grow and try new things. Success comes from learning from your mistakes, and mistakes come from trying, failing, adjusting, and trying again.

Try to change your relationship to the idea of failure and think of it as a necessary step to gain feedback and bring you closer to success.

No one is a master the first time they try something. It takes failing, often many times, to build skillsets, resilience, and a master's mindset.

If you are living in alignment with your values, then the journey of life can feel successful, regardless of what goals you achieve and what you don't. If you are living out of alignment with your own values, you will not feel good for long, no matter what you do.

"The person who has never failed has never tried."

The Shift. Own your emotions; Own your life.

Why does it take us so long sometimes to figure this out and decide to make a change? Well, for one thing, the majority of humans still do not do this.

We are bombarded with institutionalized ideas and memes and convenient social norms that invite us to belong ourselves to mediocrity, and be satisfied with being 'okay' or 'fine'.

'Good' is the enemy of 'great', but many of us struggle to even reach a threshold of feeling 'almost okay' in our modern age.

As it turns out, many of us were not given the roadmap, guidelines, or skillsets we need to keep ourselves healthy and vibrant in our current 'climates.'

It's not our fault, but it is still our responsibility.

In fact, for many of us, it does seem like the odds are stacked against us sometimes, or maybe even a lot of the time. It really doesn't matter if they are or aren't. **It is how we respond to the circumstances in life that determines the quality of our lives.**

If you find yourself stuck in a self-defeating thought loop about how you weren't dealt a great hand in life, or how such-and-such or so-&-so caused you to feel unfairly disadvantaged, then you are much like most humans who have ever been alive. See if you can get beyond that. Set that aside and ask yourself:

So what?

Now what?

Imagine you could do anything you want to with your life.

What do you really want to do?

The Purpose of Goal Setting

"If it's your job to eat a frog, it's best to do it first thing in the morning. And if it's your job to eat two frogs, it's best to eat the biggest one first." — Mark Twain

If you live in a chronically dysregulated state, you are likely to be distracted from really getting to know yourself and setting good goals. It might seem pointless or impossible from where you are now. Take a few minutes and imagine what goals you might set if you did have time to dream and make them come true.

The truth is, many of those dreams are very unlikely to come true if you are not working on them regularly. They are 100% guaranteed not to come true if you never set them.

This is really the main reason that learning to regulate your emotions and raise your emotional state is so important to living a life you love. This is why I started with the invitation to decide to take responsibility for your own life.

"If you don't write down your goals, you'll probably end up working for someone who has." — Peter Sage

We've all heard that it's important to set goals. You may not be aware that only a few people in an average cross-section of humanity actually write down and review their goals.

Those who do write down their goals and get specific about them are overwhelmingly more successful at achieving them than those who simply state them or perhaps merely keep some vague idea like "a good life" or "a happy family."

The Shift. Own your emotions; Own your life.

Without clear, specific outcomes, milestones, checkpoints, strategies, and steps, your goals are likely to remain vague dreams in the distant future. Your goals could end up always moving just out of reach.

For many, especially as aging takes its toll, goals feel like they are pulling farther and farther away. If you don't make time to write them down and regularly revisit them, they might just feel more and more distant, until eventually you find yourself giving up on them, one by one or in big swaths.

"Being fit? That was a silly dream."
"Financial security? What a fool I've been to believe I could have what everyone wants just by doing the same things that most everyone does (which is not much in the way of taking specific action to achieve my dreams)."

The point of setting goals, however, is not merely to achieve the goals. In fact, whether or not you achieve them might not even matter. **Ultimately, setting and pursuing goals is less about what you achieve and more about becoming the type of person you want to be.**

The point of having goals is to keep your 'ant' and your 'elephant' moving in the same general direction, working together, rather than spinning your wheels in self-sabotage and internal conflict.

This might seem a bit tricky to navigate, so let's dive a bit deeper into how and why to create clear goals and make revisiting them part of your regular routine.

SMARTRRR Goals

The SMART acronym is a popular framework for goal setting, especially in business circles. I add "RRR" to the end to playfully represent and highlight the very important point that goal setting is about the process of who you become in achieving them. The goals themselves are just endpoints where we reflect, reset, and repeat the entire SMART process. SMARTRRR goals are

Specific—The more specific, the better. Break it down into specific steps too if you can.

Measurable—Good goals are measurable, not vague. For example, rather than saying you are going to "improve your emotional resilience", find a way of quantifying, measuring, and charting it, such as reducing the number of times you feel triggered or have an emotional outburst over the course of a week.

Actionable—Good goals are things you can actually DO. In our example of improving emotional resilience, this needs to be paired with an action, such as "by meditating every day for at least ten minutes and journaling before bed every night".

Realistic—Good goals should be in that sweet spot of 'just challenging enough', but not so challenging you won't do them. Challenge yourself but don't set yourself up for failure. Set goals that are just a little bit past your comfort zone.

Timebound—Good goals have a deadline or time element. Even if your goal is something ongoing or long-term, break it down into incremental steps and assign a check point and a threshold you think you can achieve.

Again, I propose we add another aspect to the goal setting process upfront and plan for a period to **Reflect, Reset, and Repeat** the process.

Reflecting on our goals and on our progress is a crucial step in effective goal setting. Remember, the goal is more about becoming the type of person you want to become than accomplishing the goal itself. It is important to reflect on what worked and what didn't. Reflect on what surprised you, what challenged you, what felt easy, and what was effective; whether you succeed in achieving your goal or not.

Then be sure to **adjust and reset** either an updated version of your goal or a different goal and **repeat the entire process**.

This goes on until...pretty much forever—which is why it is super important that you choose goals you can enjoy accomplishing or trying to accomplish along the way.

If you find a goal is not moving you towards the person you want to become, that's okay. Reflect on why and make adjustments based on the feedback you get, from yourself and from others.

Setting the Bar Just Right

Good goals should feel just barely attainable or slightly out of reach, at least at first. If you can easily see how to reach your goals when you set them, then they are not goals that will lead you to develop yourself very much. Setting good goals is a skill you can develop with practice.

You need to have at least one or two big goals that are outside your comfort zone and at least a little bit beyond your current reach.

Of course, you do want to be able to achieve your goals. Just be mindful that there is a 'sweet spot' for goals that is not too easy and not too difficult. Also keep in mind that you will need to set new goals along the way, to keep yourself evolving, consciously.

If you find yourself feeling discouraged because you are not reaching your goals, then lower the bar a bit, or give yourself some 'bumper rails'. Look at the section on neurochemistry and see if you can identify any patterns you might be able to fix with a slight adjustment to your reward system, once you are more aware of what is driving you and what is getting in your way.

If you find yourself feeling uninspired or unfocused, you might need to raise the bar a bit and see if you can rev up or rally some extra zig and impress yourself with your own progress.

You might be surprised at what you can do when you really challenge yourself. It is also totally fine to make the bar 'just' showing up and staying in the room, doing the work, developing better habits. That's a lot!

Keep in mind, there is no 'normal' path or rate of speed you should be developing into yourself. There is not one 'right way' to live a good life. Your life story is yours to create.

The Shift. Own your emotions; Own your life.

On some level this process never ends, and you can't get it wrong. This process can be slower or faster though, and more or less enjoyable and fulfilling.

If it feels wrong then it's either just not familiar yet because it is new, or it is out of alignment with your values and/or beliefs. Over time and with practice you will get better at discerning the difference and learn to make evaluating and adjusting your goals and your progress a regular practice.

Remember, the object of these big goals is to motivate your own progress and self-development. **At the end of the day, and at the end of your lifetime, it is how you feel about yourself when you are by yourself that matters most, not which goals you achieved and which you didn't.**

That does not mean you should set your sights on things you don't believe are possible. It does mean that you don't need to be able to see all the steps to take the first one. It means you don't need to set goals that have a clear path to success but rather set goals that lead you to become the person you want to be.

Studies have shown that we humans do best when we set a goal that we believe is in reach, much better than when we believe the goal is out of reach. When a goal seems out of reach, or if it is too easy, we often stop trying.

When we just have to do a little bit more (somewhere around 4%-20%), we succeed in reaching that more often. Once we find the new goal is coming easily, then we can set the bar a little bit higher.

The Shift. Own your emotions; Own your life.

If we have a larger goal, one that seems hard, like a very high mountain to climb, it can be helpful to plan a reward for ourselves to help give ourselves a little extra motivation. The green bars work well enough on my step counting app, for example, but the larger goal of feeling fit enough to enjoy the upcoming snowboarding season needs a bit more than green bars to get me doing those extra strengthening exercises. For that, I use the incentive of buying myself a season pass for snowboarding.

For super big goals, like writing and publishing this book, I use even bigger rewards and incentives to help motivate myself and keep myself on track.

My reward for finishing this book will be a tandem skydiving trip. Of course, finishing and publishing the book is a reward in and of itself, but the extra incentive of planning a trip to check off another exciting item on my 'bucket list' helps give me extra motivation on those days when life offers to take up all my time on so many little things. It adds weight to the goal and helps me prioritize it more enthusiastically.

➤ **INVITATION TO ACTION:** Think about a goal you have for yourself, and brainstorm ways you can pump up more motivation for yourself to accomplish it. Maybe that is breaking it down into smaller steps. Maybe that is stacking it in with other goals, so it gets more of your time and energy. Maybe it's adding an extra incentive or reward for yourself when you accomplish it. Maybe it is some combination of all three of these.

The Shift. Own your emotions; Own your life.

Remember, there is not one right way to do this. The key is to figure out what works best for you and do more of that. Also keep in mind that what motivates you is likely to change over time, and so will your goals. Make goal-setting a regular part of your routine or habit stack for best results.

I think it is worth considering that our sense of self-worth seems to be greatly enhanced by attempting and at least occasionally achieving success when doing 'hard things.'

Consider a goal like 'climbing a high mountain' or 'making it off the highest lift and down the mountain without falling down.' You might be pursuing a goal like getting a degree, raising healthy, happy children, publishing a best-selling book, or recording and producing an LP of original music.

Having goals is important and can help drive improvements. However, once one is accomplished, you will need a new goal.

Goals are important and also somewhat arbitrary. It isn't actually a specific goal that makes attaining it worthwhile. If we do this right, it is the neurochemistry we get along the way.

The real purpose of achieving goals is the feeling of being the type of person who achieves their goals. It is knowing you did it, not the actuality of having done it, at least in most cases.

Many of us didn't receive the foundation of healthy, secure attachments to loving parents, grandparents, and extended family members. Some of us were born into poverty; others into the sterile, unloving environment that can accompany extreme wealth. It's a beautiful part of this life that we all

The Shift. Own your emotions; Own your life.

have our own, unique life stories. Be sure to set goals that suit your own story and where you are on your own unique journey.

If you ever find yourself feeling like it is all futile, and there is no point in pursuing goals that you feel you can't accomplish, you are not alone. I feel this way often, and I also know that things can always get better or worse. Our chemical-laden environments and food supplies may make it increasingly difficult to be born into and maintain a fully functioning, healthy body.

While this might seem frightening at times, it can also be a great motivator. None of this is a reason to give up or to not try to create a more vibrant life. Many incredible people have come and gone before us and their life stories can be a beautiful reminder that the point of life is not to live the same story as anyone else. The point of your life is to live your story, the best that you can.

Our time here is finite. All this is temporary. So, go out and get some life on you, for goodness' sake! Embracing change and taking charge of your life is the path to true fulfillment, even if it's not always comfortable. Remember, we are all in this together, and no other human has perfected being you like you--and only you--can.

"Constant change is afoot. Comfort is still two socks." —GAL

Put the Big Rocks in First

A story about priorities:

Some years ago, I attended a weekend seminar on qi gong. The instructor was a prestigious man from China. He had trained in many fields, including qi gong, kung fu, and ninjutsu.

He was a special guest at a ninjutsu school I belonged to at the time. He was traveling the U.S., promoting several books and videos he had authored and published, and our school invited him to promote his instructional goods and expand our knowledge of moving meditations such as qi gong/tai chi. He lectured us on the importance of discipline and consistency, and also focused on the basics of correct posture, balance, and breathing.

He had many stories from being a world traveler and a life-long student of martial arts. By our second day with him, we were all impressed and humbled by his achievements and his ability to hold our attention and cultivate so much respect, despite being from a different culture and at least two decades older than the oldest among us.

He was lecturing us on the importance of meditation and breathing techniques, and he stated that he spent 2–3 hours every day in seated meditation, plus another couple of hours in moving meditation.

We were all aware that he had flown from the east coast to host our weekend seminar while still maintaining authority at a school where he was a regular instructor, and of course, creating more than a dozen videos and books. This was back before the days of print on demand or (believe it or not) even the internet.

The Shift. Own your emotions; Own your life.

Someone finally got up the courage to question him. "Do you really spend that much time EVERY day? I mean, even when you are traveling? How is that even possible?"

He smiled and said, "Yes. Especially when I am traveling. I make sure I take care of my energy first. That is the only way I can keep doing all the things I do."

"But how?" the student asked. "I mean, there are only so many hours in a day. It doesn't seem possible to spend 4–5 hours every day meditating and doing tai chi, just working on your energy and still get any actual work done or have a life--let alone run a school, make videos, and write books--not to mention traveling..."

He smiled, took a deep breath, and sat down on the floor in front of us.

"You stay in horse stance," he said, as a few of us started to contemplate sitting down as well.

"I will tell you a story while you work. I did not come here to watch you not work."

So we stood in horse stance, some of us with legs already beginning to shake, and he proceeded.

"Tuck your butt," he said, still smiling calmly. This was an instruction he had already repeated countless times and would continue to repeat throughout our time together.

"Remember to breathe."

He took a deep breath himself and then told us this story:

"A long time ago, I had an instructor who was doing so many things, and I was like you, not understanding how he could do so many things and still be such a master of his own art. Someone asked him, just like you asked me, 'How do you do it?'

Our instructor smiled again and took another deep, slow breath and exhaled audibly and we exhaled with him.

"The next day, our instructor brought a pitcher of water, a jar, and a box with several things in it and set them up on a table in front of us. He took out several rocks from his box and put them in the jar until he could not fit any more rocks inside. 'Now,' he said, 'tell me, is this jar full?' Several of us nodded our heads, and a couple of people said, 'Yes, it appears to be full.'

The master then took out a bowl from the box and began to drop pebbles from the bowl into the jar. They fell in between the rocks. When he had put in so many that the pebbles began to spill onto the table, he asked us again, 'Now, what do you think? Is it full?' We were less confident, and only a couple of us nodded our heads.

The master pulled out a bag of sand from the box and poured the sand into the jar, filling the spaces between the rocks and the pebbles. Finally, the sand began to spill onto the table. He tapped the jar and put in a little more. Again, he asked us, 'Is it full now?' A few more students nodded this time, and a couple said 'yes' again.

The master then poured the water from the pitcher into the jar. 'Now it is full,' he said. 'Always remember, you must put the big rocks in first.'"

I think of this story often when I'm feeling overwhelmed or like I cannot do all the things I want to do. It's easy to get caught up in mundane tasks, those little things that are like grains of sand or pebbles.

The Shift. Own your emotions; Own your life.

To get the really important things done in life, you need to prioritize what is most important and make sure those things get done before you worry about the smaller, less significant tasks. You will need to learn to say "no" to a lot of things.

This also reminds me of the famous quote attributed to Mark Twain: "If you must eat a frog, eat it first thing in the morning. And if you must eat two frogs, eat the biggest one first."

What does this story make you think of?

Are there big rocks in your life that you are running out of room for because you keep filling your time with smaller, less significant things?

Are you telling yourself a story that you don't have time to take care of your health or your most important relationships because you must take care of so many mundane tasks first?

Do you spend your time repeating insignificant or even unhealthy actions at the expense of the things you truly want in your life?

I also think it's important to evaluate the general quality of all the different-sized 'rocks' we are filling our time with. Without conscious choosing, we could end up eating various-sized frogs all day instead of enjoying delicious salads and, yes, even cookies sometimes.

Make sure you are putting in the right rocks...

Many human lives, including mine, are largely filled with little and sometimes large things we don't really like or that do not make us feel like the people we want to be.

The Shift. Own your emotions; Own your life.

This is why I choose to do jobs that are better suited for me. It's a big part of why I no longer watch the "news" or any programming that makes me feel bad or unconscious for very long. It's just not who I want to be; not how I want to focus my energy and attention. It's why I choose healthier cookies.

It's important to point out that there is not one 'right way' to be. It's a beautiful thing that we are all unique, and it would be dismal if we all liked the same 'rocks' or wanted the details of our lives to be exactly the same.

Having your own style and preferences is a wonderful aspect of living and should be celebrated. It's important to reflect on what that means to you and to give yourself permission to change your mind, change your style, and rearrange the furniture from time to time. I'm talking to myself here as much as anyone else.

A great life is not full of just any 'rocks'; it's full of big rocks, pebbles, grains of sand, and water (to use the metaphors from the story I mentioned). But if we don't pay attention to each of those and make sure to choose those that are aligned with the type of person we want to be, we could end up in jobs we hate, relationships that are not healthy, eating 'frogs' for breakfast regularly when we don't even really prefer to eat frogs at all.

It's also worth mentioning that you can prefer something—frogs or no frogs—chocolate or vanilla—without wanting to destroy or hating what you don't prefer. Simply choose what you prefer and say "no thanks, not today" to what you do not prefer.

There is no need to go out of your way to avoid what you do not want. You don't have to make it an enemy. Simply

123

The Shift. Own your emotions; Own your life.

choose more of what you do want and you will naturally get less of what you don't want.

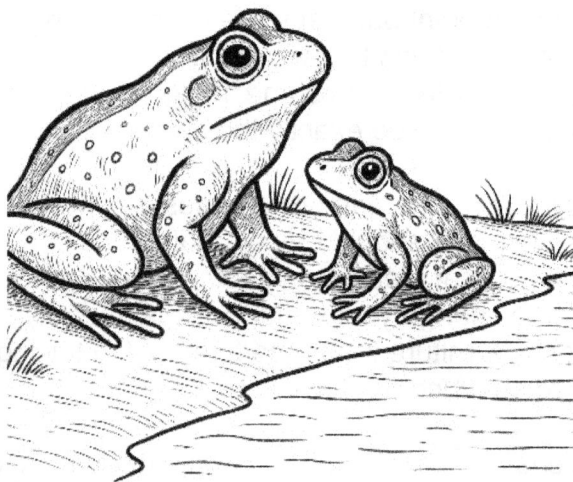

The Power of Taking Responsibility

Taking responsibility for our actions, emotions, and circumstances is the foundation of personal growth and self-mastery. It's about recognizing that we are in the driver's seat of our own lives--not waiting for someone else to change things or blaming outside forces.

Research consistently shows that when we take ownership of our lives, we experience more emotional resilience, confidence, and mental well-being. By embracing this responsibility, we reclaim our power to shape the outcomes we desire.

Studies confirm that individuals with an internal locus of control--the belief that they have the power to influence their own live--report higher life satisfaction and greater mental health. Those who see themselves as responsible for their circumstances tend to take proactive steps toward positive change.

On the flip side, those with an external locus of control, who blame circumstances or others for their problems, often feel stuck and powerless. Owning your choices, your emotions, and your life opens the door to empowerment, motivation, and emotional mastery.

There's also research to support that taking responsibility leads to higher self-esteem and greater success in all areas of life. At least one study found that when people own their decisions and behavior, they experience better problem-solving abilities and more personal success. Why? Because they're not waiting for permission or for someone else to fix things--they're stepping up, taking action, and making things happen.

The self-determination theory (SDT), developed by psychologists Edward Deci and Richard Ryan, underscores that when we experience a sense of autonomy, we feel more ownership over our choices, which is essential for emotional well-being. When we take responsibility, we're claiming our autonomy, our ability to shape our own path— and with that comes greater emotional health, competence, and fulfillment.

The American Psychological Association also highlights the connection between personal accountability and emotional regulation. Studies have found that people who take responsibility for their own emotional states--who say, "I own this, I can change this"--are better equipped to manage stress, handle challenges, and grow emotionally. Instead of reacting to life, they respond to it. That's the real key to self-mastery--choosing to be in charge of your own emotional landscape and being able to control your emotional state.

Really, you probably don't need me or anyone else to convince you, if you are honest with yourself. Most of us know the positive feelings that come from feeling like we are in control of our lives and making positive strides, vs. how it feels when we are just blaming others or wallowing in shame and feeling like there is no way out, and no hope for change.

The truth is, even if hope seems to disappear sometimes, in my experience, hope always returns. It returns faster sometimes when we take responsibility for our own lives.

The Shift. Own your emotions; Own your life.

Regaining hope requires us to get moving and take some positive action to stir up stagnation and disrupt dysfunctional patterns.

Many of us know all this but we still think "yeah but…" or "not me though, because I am too (fill in the blank)" or "easy for you to say, you don't know what I am going through".

Of course I don't know what you are going through. I have no doubt you have gone through a lot. We all do. Yes, some more than others, but no one gets through life without some suffering, even if it is simply from that existential dread that plagues us from time to time with the knowing that no one gets out alive.

What you are going through matters. Your feelings are valid. And also, none of it is a good reason not to decide to take responsibility for your own life and get more emotionally fit so you can improve your chances to really create a life you love.

It's About the Process, Not the Destination

Progress is not a straight line, nor is it a final destination. Instead, it's an ongoing journey shaped by the choices we make and the course corrections we take along the way. The key is to enjoy the ride while continuously checking your internal compass to ensure you're headed in the right direction.

The Shift. Own your emotions; Own your life.

One of my favorite online teachers and coaches, Tom Bilyeu, frequently speaks about applying the scientific method to move forward, whether in business or personal development. He emphasizes that while failure is guaranteed, success is not.

This is where the growth mindset becomes essential. We must learn to see failure not as an endpoint but as a form of feedback. Failure is a critical step along the path of progress.

Much like developing a hypothesis (based on observations) and then testing it through experimentation with the scientific method to develop working theories, life requires us to test our goals and decisions. We try new things, assess how well they align with our values and aspirations, and adjust accordingly.

Embracing failure as feedback helps us refine our process. It's not about being 'right' or 'wrong'; instead, think of it as "slow progress" versus "faster progress." Sometimes it's the "cha cha cha" (two steps forward, one step back).

Innovation and real 'quantum leaps' often happen only through seemingly catastrophic failures or feeling like we have no other option. Failure doesn't have to be catastrophic though. In fact, mastery requires that we fail often and rarely catastrophically.

We ought to try to fail forward; learn from our mistakes, adjust, and fail again. We must at least be willing to fail, to try things we are not sure will succeed sometimes, in order to find out where our limits really are.

Pictures or it didn't happen

Another important component is to track your progress. By keeping track of what is working and what is not you can continuously refine your toolkit and increase the efficiency and effectiveness of your efforts. You will also be building a body of evidence of your own personal growth which you can reflect on and use to help cultivate a positive, growth-focused mindset.

This mindset is especially important when learning to listen to and regulate your emotions. Just as you would test a hypothesis and gather data in an experiment, you need to test your emotional responses and gauge how well they serve you. To make any meaning out of all this data, you need to write it down, organize it, track it, review it, and adjust your strategies from time to time.

At times, you may react poorly, misjudge a situation, or make decisions that don't align with your best self. These moments aren't setbacks--they're opportunities to recalibrate, refine your emotional toolkit, and grow. The very practice of noticing these moments and then deciding to learn and grow from them--deciding to tell a better story, be more compassionate and patient with yourself--is worth celebrating.

When you track your emotions, your habits and your outcomes, they become data points that you can work with to improve your life, instead of just evidence you use against yourself as reasons you don't have the life you want.

The Shift. Own your emotions; Own your life.

What's crucial here is maintaining humility. You will be wrong more often than you will be 'right,' and that's okay. In fact, you should expect it. The beauty of the process is that progress is not about perfection--it's about continuous improvement.

You may stumble or falter, but each misstep is another opportunity to adjust your path. As long as you're willing to course-correct and learn from the data--your failures, feedback, and emotions--you will move forward.

It's also essential to remember that real growth happens through friction and challenge. In physics, objects at rest tend to stay at rest, and motion only begins when a force is applied. In the same way, the act of striving toward change inherently invites resistance--whether it's internal (self-doubt, fear, bad habits) or external (circumstances, obstacles).

Just as friction strengthens muscle, it also strengthens character. Without resistance, there can be no real growth.

Momentum is your friend--IF you are heading in the right direction. Once you've taken that first step, breaking through inertia, you will find that progress becomes easier.

Just as objects in motion tend to stay in motion, your actions--no matter how small--will gather speed and create the momentum necessary for personal transformation.

Of course, it is important to ensure that your efforts and the momentum you are building are aligned with your goals. Just like in physics, where force must be applied in the right direction to produce meaningful movement, your goals and actions must be aligned with your deeper values.

The Shift. Own your emotions; Own your life.

Otherwise, all your effort may feel like wasted energy, driving you in circles or even backwards rather than toward real fulfillment. This alignment between your actions and your purpose is the foundation for lasting, meaningful progress.

Summary of Chapter Three

Get ready to let go of old patterns and baggage that no longer serve you. You can just set that stuff down right here.

Now that we've covered some basic definitions and you are armed with essential questions and the decision to become the master of your own emotions and destiny, we are ready to dive deeper into the tools you can use to help you develop a more coherent, less overwhelmed life.

Put down your worries and firmly-held beliefs about your limitations, even if it is just for a while. If you can't quite do that yet, try to imagine what it might feel like to put them down--suspend them temporarily, just for now. What might it feel like if you COULD put them down? Allow yourself to imagine it, even if it's just for a little while. You can always pick them back up if you find they are serving you.

In my experience, life offers a constant stream of things we can fret about, worry over, and feel slighted by, just as it also offers a constant stream of delights. It is up to us to choose what we will highlight as the decorative details of our lives. I urge you to try it. What have you got to lose?

An important aspect of this journey is learning when to let go and when to hold on. Our aim is to develop clear and strong convictions that we hold loosely.

The Shift. Own your emotions; Own your life.

It will be scary at times; I do know. I have learned that when it becomes apparent that it is time to grow--time to shed your old skin, release the old and busted beliefs, sayings, and things that no longer serve you--it's best to relax, bend your knees a little, trust yourself, exhale, and let go of the past like it was yesterday. Holding on beyond the time something serves your progress will only slow down your inevitable growth, and it could also break off a fingernail or two.

Keep your courage close, and remember that feeling uncomfortable or even wildly uncertain sometimes is a natural part of this process. To desire to have no struggles and no discomfort is unrealistic for living a dynamic life. True living is messy.

Take heart in knowing it will be temporary, and as you practice this Shift, it will become easier and more natural. The gaps will become less uncomfortable until such time as you have grown so much that you are ready to transform again.

Just like working out at the gym can gradually increase your strength and eventually make what was hard seem easy, emotional fitness and learning to master your brain and the rest of your nervous system will get easier with practice.

It is also important to remember that things happen in waves, in cycles, and it is natural for everything to ebb and flow to some extent. My mission here is to help you learn to 'ride the waves' of these cycles, ideally with some style and grace, while finding more joy and fulfillment in living your beautiful life.

The Shift. Own your emotions; Own your life.

INVITATION TO ACTION: Take out some paper and make a list of all the things you do in a typical week. Then make a list of the things you would like to accomplish or do. Are the things you are doing regularly supporting your goals, closing the gaps, or are they driving you farther from them, day by day? Be honest with yourself.

Spend some time contemplating everything you are filling your time with and ask yourself if it is moving you closer or farther away from the person you think you want to be.

Then write down at least one small change you can make today, and take at least one action, which you will be glad you did tomorrow.

Real People Who Inspire Me:

Simone Giertz: Embracing Imperfection and Joyful Creativity

Simone Giertz, known as the "Queen of Shitty Robots," has inspired millions with her unique blend of humor, creativity, and resilience. Her story is a testament to the power of embracing imperfection and turning failures into fun, innovative solutions.

Starting as an inventor of intentionally ridiculous robots, Simone quickly became a YouTube sensation, challenging the notion that success must come from polished perfection.

Her journey took a more profound turn when she was diagnosed with a brain tumor. During her recovery, Simone confronted her vulnerabilities and reconnected with the deeper joy of creation.

This transformation shifted her focus from comedy to meaningful design projects, such as building her dream camper and launching a quirky yet practical product line.

Throughout her work, Simone embodies the archetype of the Creator, showing that the process of making--even when messy--can be an act of healing and self-expression.

Tererai Trent: Planting Dreams and Growing Hope

Tererai Trent's journey began in a small village in Zimbabwe, where cultural expectations limited girls' opportunities to pursue education. Married off at a young age and raising children before she had the chance to realize her own potential, Tererai's dream of getting an education seemed out of reach. But she refused to let her circumstances define her future.

As a young girl with unwavering determination, Tererai wrote down her dreams on a piece of paper--to study in the United States, earn a bachelor's, master's, and PhD--and buried them in a tin can under a rock, symbolizing her commitment to turning those dreams into reality.

Over the years, Tererai faced countless obstacles, from financial hardship to cultural expectations that told her women could never achieve such lofty goals.

She leaned on the power of visualization, persistence, and community support, and in an incredible story of relentless pursuit of her dreams, Tererai eventually earned scholarships to study in the U.S.

A pivotal moment came when Oprah Winfrey heard her story and became an ally in her journey, providing funding and a platform to help Tererai realize her vision. Even as she pursued her education, she never forgot her roots, vowing to give back to her community.

With Oprah's support, Tererai returned to Zimbabwe to build schools and create opportunities for countless children. Last time I checked, she was living in Santa Fe, New Mexico.

Tererai now spends her energy empowering other women to follow their own dreams. Her story is a powerful testament to the ripple effect of one person's determination: by achieving her own dreams, she has inspired generations of students to dream big and believe in their potential.

Codie Sanchez: Turning Struggles into Strategic Success

Codie Sanchez is a force of nature in the world of finance and entrepreneurship, known for her ability to transform overlooked opportunities into thriving ventures. Growing up as a Latina in a predominantly white, male-dominated industry, Codie often felt underestimated and out of place. Instead of letting these challenges discourage her, she used them as motivation to prove her worth and carve out her own path.

Early in her career, Codie worked as a journalist covering human rights abuses, where she witnessed unimaginable struggles and resilience. These experiences shaped her perspective on the power of small, consistent actions to create change.

Later, she pivoted into finance, becoming a leader in private equity and launching her own businesses focused on buying and growing "boring" small businesses--an unconventional approach that has inspired a new generation of entrepreneurs.

The Shift. Own your emotions; Own your life.

Codie's success is rooted in habits like relentless learning, strategic thinking, and the courage to challenge the status quo. She shares her insights widely, empowering others to think differently about wealth creation and build legacies that last. Her story demonstrates that even the smallest steps--like questioning assumptions or seeking untapped potential--can lead to quantum leaps in impact.

Richard Branson: Living Boldly and Innovating Fearlessly

Richard Branson, the iconic founder of Virgin Group, is synonymous with bold ambition and innovation. He has inspired me for decades now and continues to bring innovation and style to his businesses.

Many people don't know that he is severely dyslexic and was often dismissed in school. Branson struggled with traditional education but discovered his strengths in creativity and entrepreneurship.

He launched his first business, a student magazine, at the age of 16 and soon moved into the music industry, founding Virgin Records. Despite initial skepticism, he built one of the most successful record labels of the era, signing groundbreaking artists and challenging the status quo.

Believe it or not, Branson's journey hasn't been without major setbacks. From failed ventures to near-catastrophic financial crises, he's faced countless obstacles that tested his resilience. Yet, his approach to failure--viewing it as a stepping stone to success--has been instrumental in his growth.

The Shift. Own your emotions; Own your life.

Branson relies on habits like visualization, risk assessment, and cultivating a positive mindset to navigate challenges. He's also a firm believer in surrounding himself with a strong team, emphasizing the importance of collaboration and shared goals.

Beyond his business empire, Branson's commitment to philanthropy and environmental sustainability demonstrates his belief in creating lasting, positive change. Through initiatives like Virgin Unite, he's leveraged his resources to tackle global challenges, proving that entrepreneurship can be a force for good. His story inspires me to dream big, embrace failure, and take bold steps toward building a better world.

Simone Giertz, Tererai Trent, Codie Sanchez, and Richard Branson each exemplify the principles of personal responsibility and utilizing atomic habits and quantum leaps in unique ways. Each turned their struggles into sources of strength, using consistent effort and strategic vision to achieve their goals and create lasting systemic change.

Their stories remind us that even the most daunting challenges can be opportunities to grow, innovate, and inspire others.

By planting dreams, taking bold actions, and staying committed to their values, they've created ripples of positive change that will continue to reverberate for generations to come. Their legacies are a call to action for all of us to dream big, take consistent steps, and create a better world.

The Shift. Own your emotions; Own your life.

The Scorpion and the Frog

One intense monsoon day, the river swelled and rushed along its banks rapidly. A scorpion found itself stranded, unable to cross. He was trapped by the fast-moving waters and knew he couldn't swim. Desperate, he spotted a frog preparing to leap into the river and called out to him.

"Frog, would you be so kind as to carry me across the river on your back? I cannot swim, and without your help, I will surely be stuck here."

The frog, wary and wise, eyed the scorpion cautiously. "I would help you," said the frog, "but you are a scorpion. If I carry you on my back, what's to stop you from stinging me?"

The scorpion smiled reassuringly. "Oh, you need not worry. If I were to sting you, we would both drown. Surely I wouldn't do something so foolish. It would be against my own interest. I promise I will not sting you if you carry me across."

The Shift. Own your emotions; Own your life.

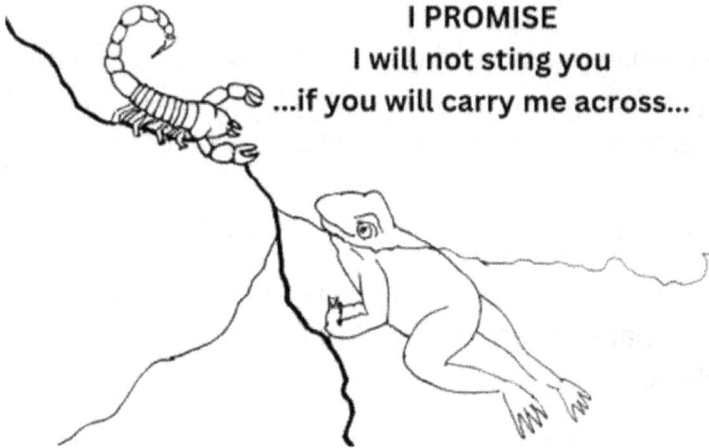

I PROMISE
I will not sting you
...if you will carry me across...

The frog thought about this and reasoned that the scorpion had a point. If the scorpion were to sting him, they would both perish in the river. Trusting the logic, the frog agreed and let the scorpion climb onto his back. Then, together, they set out across the water.

For a time, they traveled smoothly, the frog's powerful legs propelling them forward. But as they reached the middle of the river, the frog felt a sharp, searing pain in his back. The scorpion had stung him.

The frog, shocked and dying, cried out, "Why? Why did you sting me? Now we'll both die!"

As the waters began to swirl around them, the scorpion replied with a somber finality, "I couldn't help it. It's in my nature."

CHAPTER 4
"QUIT HITTING YOURSELF"
— Why we self-sabotage and how to stop it.

You are making things harder than they have to be.

It's not just you though. Nearly all of us do this. We sabotage our own efforts more often than anything else does, and often we are bewildered about why we keep doing the same, self-defeating things; making the same suboptimal choices and engaging in the same unhealthy habits.

Why do we self-sabotage?

The short answer is that we do it to fill some need. We do it out of habit. We do it out of misdirection or for distraction. We do it for security, predictability, and pattern recognition. Sometimes, we do it for novelty, love, or external and internal validation. It can be complicated.

We are complex social creatures having complex biological experiences. Often, we are using strategies that were the best we could come up with earlier in life. Some of them may have even served us very well at a time, but eventually, most of our strategies need updating or they can become limiting.

Self-sabotage can take many forms--procrastination, addiction, avoidance, or negative self-talk. We may know that these behaviors harm us, yet we continue to engage in them, often feeling bewildered or frustrated because we don't understand why.

The first step to breaking these patterns is to recognize them, to understand where our actions originate and why we continue to engage in them. This awareness allows us to begin the process of change, of transforming our "nature" into something that serves us rather than sabotages us.

Understanding what underlying need we are trying to fill with any self-sabotaging behavior can be the key to growing past it. Once we know what need we are trying to meet, we can find healthier ways of meeting that need. We can stop spending our time and energy on behaviors that no longer serve us.

Many books have been written about how we meet our basic needs. Maslow's hierarchy of needs, published some 80 years ago, remains one of the key frameworks even though many people still do not have most of these needs met.

I don't completely agree that these are in the exact hierarchy that he posed. In my experience, sometimes a lack of basic needs can result in a transcendent experience that sometimes leads to a leap in self-awareness and more self-actualization. Nonetheless, this can be a helpful framework to consider what might be motivating you to engage in self-sabotaging behaviors.

The Shift. Own your emotions; Own your life.

If your body is responding to feeling unsafe, the first order of business is to re-regulate your nervous system. As long as you are dysregulated, you can work on improving your level of emotional fitness.

To review, Maslow's hierarchy of needs are:

Physiological needs: the basics--food, water, shelter, clothing, and sleep. Sadly, a significant number of people either lack these essentials or have them met inadequately. Many of us have access to having these met and still manage to falter when it comes to taking good care of these basic needs. We don't get enough sleep. We don't eat nourishing meals or drink clean water. We bombard ourselves with toxic inputs such as processed food, junk entertainment, and self-limiting thoughts. We overwork ourselves and deny ourselves the recovery time and healing touch we need to thrive, and then we wonder why we are having a hard time. It's important to take a look at how well you are meeting your own basic needs and adjust as needed, especially if you are chronically dysregulated.

Safety and security: this includes some level of predictability. Many of us strive to create a sense of safety and security through predictability, even if it isn't entirely pleasant or healthy. In times of rapid change, we often crave some sense of familiarity so much that we will tolerate or even crave abuse or maltreatment, listen to the same songs over and over, eat the same crappy meals every day, and think the same repeating self-defeating or limiting thoughts just to give ourselves some sense of security.

Love and belonging: many of us don't have this need met from early on. In response, we often develop unhealthy patterns to cope. We may align ourselves with outcasts or unhealthy habits, seeking external validation in all sorts of harmful ways. Some find a sense of belonging in addictive patterns with food, drugs, television, or other unhealthy habits. One of my favorite books *Belonging: Remembering Ourselves Home*, by Toko-pa Turner, beautifully illustrates how we can find that sense of belonging in healthier ways, by building healthy communities and by remembering that we are earthlings, who naturally belong to and on this planet.

Self-esteem: next comes self-esteem, or feeling a sense of self-worth, at least according to Maslow. I am not entirely convinced about the hierarchical order of these needs, but I do think they are worth evaluating and reflecting on how well we are meeting each of these. In Maslow's model, Self-esteem is followed by

Self-actualization at the top of the hierarchy. This is becoming your fullest, truest self, and what we are really aiming at here. It is difficult to pursue self-esteem and self-actualization if your more basic needs are not met adequately--though I also think that sometimes improving our self-esteem and sense of self-actualization can help motivate us to take better care of those needs considered lower on Maslow's hierarchy.

Another reason we might self-sabotage is that humans often love doing hard things. Perhaps because it builds strength and adds to our sense of accomplishment. Maybe we believe it's tied to our value or worthiness. Perhaps it feeds our self-esteem.

It's important to consciously examine our actions. Our behaviors and efforts need to be aligned with our values. This requires understanding what our values are.

The Shift. Own your emotions; Own your life.

Knowing your values is key to getting back to a more regulated state. Living out of alignment with your values will lead to feelings of discordance and incoherence.

INVITATION TO ACTION: I invite you to take a few minutes now to think about what your own personal values are. Write down the things you value most. Is it honesty? Creativity? Stability? Family? Remember, there is no 'right answer' and it is a beautiful aspect of humanity that our values vary. You might have a long list, but try to narrow it down to your top 3–5.

Right now, mine are creativity, curiosity, courage, and authenticity. Everyone's values will differ, and that's part of our uniqueness. Values can change over time, although they tend to be long-lasting. It's a beautiful aspect of humanity that we care deeply about different things, and also, there are many similarities in most of our values.

Take some time to reflect on your values and become conscious of them. Then, reflect on your actions and see if your day-to-day behaviors support or hinder your alignment with these values.

This exercise should be done regularly. It's a good idea to reflect on your values daily or weekly, at least briefly.

Consider doing a deeper self-inquiry monthly, seasonally, or at least once a year. Your top values might change over time, though they'll likely remain more consistent once you become clear on what they really are and why.

Incongruence with our values (and also just plain 'bad habits') is at the heart of self-sabotage. Our emotions are our bodies' way of communicating nuanced, multisensory inputs, which are then filtered through our stories, memories, words, frames, and possibilities. When the stories we tell ourselves about our emotions don't align with our values and beliefs, we experience incoherence or discordance.

How are you making things harder than they have to be?

Are you repeating self-defeating stories?

We create stories based on our 'feelings,' which then get reinterpreted by our emotional systems in a constant feedback loop. The stories we tell ourselves about the emotions and data we collect reinforce themselves.

It's important to recognize that our patterns and habits usually come from coping strategies--ours or our ancestors or those of the people around us. There are often very real, very good--or logical--reasons that we develop the self-sabotaging narratives we do.

Give yourself a little more grace and be patient with yourself. See if you can discover more about what you want and need to feel fulfilled in this life.

Another key to overcoming self-sabotage is to recognize this pattern and shift the narrative. One way to do this is by asking yourself better questions. Learn to pause when you recognize you're spiraling in a 'trauma loop,' raise your frequency, and use your dysfunction as an invitation to grow and improve. Untangle the thoughts causing incoherence in your body.

It's common to repeat self-defeating narratives like:

"No one loves me."

The Shift. Own your emotions; Own your life.

"I'm not worthy of love."

"I must be unlovable."

"I'm not good enough."

"I'm too young/old/fat/thin/tall/short/quiet/loud/stupid/smart…"

"People never do as much for me as I do for them."

"Maybe if I sacrifice a little more of myself…"

These thoughts often drag us down into the 'pit of despair.'

A quick way out is to be more honest and gentler with yourself. When you catch yourself repeating a negative thought, ask:

"Is that really true?"

"Is this the whole truth and nothing but the truth?"

"How would it be if I didn't believe this?"

"Can I find a thought that feels a bit better?"

"It is helpful to think about this right now?"

You may convince yourself that it's true, at least right now. But check in with how it feels in your body. When you're telling yourself the truth, it will feel better. If you're truly honest with yourself and approach these questions with the intention of finding the truth, you'll see that our human minds are very limited, and nothing we think is ever the 'whole truth and nothing but the truth.'

The Shift. Own your emotions; Own your life.

Disrupt the pattern.

Disruption doesn't always feel good. In fact, it often feels uncomfortable, scary, or even 'wrong' at the beginning. Growth requires letting go of old patterns and being willing to be uncomfortable in new, unfamiliar situations and mindsets.

"Don't hold on to a mistake just because you spent a long time making it."

We often repeat negative, self-defeating thoughts as a way of 'proving our limitations.' We often keep repeating the same mistakes because we feel invested in them after giving them so much time and attention. We make up stories about how our self-defeating thoughts are part of our fixed identity. If you keep doing that, it might seem more and more true.

The way out of this loop is to interrupt the pattern. Tell a different story, or at least, change your perspective on a key detail or two.

If you can't shift to a more positive or expansive thought at first, try a healthy distraction. Disrupt the pattern. Change your routine. Change your surroundings. Take a trip or rearrange your furniture. Wear a different outfit. Get a haircut or some new boots.

Yes, I know it might sound silly or futile, but a change of pattern can create an opening for you to change your perspective and your story, even if it is just a little bit at first.

Start where you are and do the best you can with what you have. Take a step in the direction of positive change, even if it is a tiny step, and even if you fail on your first, second, or third attempt.

The Shift. Own your emotions; Own your life.

Remind yourself that change can take time, and your choice to create positive change is a huge step in and of itself. Disrupting the pattern can create a little space, a little potential, and room for something lighter to come in.

Now you are in The Shift.

Here's some 'food for thought' that might be a bit of a bitter pill to swallow: we tend to project our perceptions and feelings onto others and judge, condemn, or idolize aspects of other people that we have not fully integrated and accepted as parts of ourselves.

Accepting behaviors in others is the same as accepting those behaviors in yourself on some level. Rejecting others is the same as rejecting parts of yourself on some level.

Be sure to check in with your values any time you feel critical or judgmental of anyone, including yourself. Give yourself a lot of grace when you do notice you are being critical or judgmental. You are still human after all.

There is a subtle but important distinction between accepting and loving. You can accept and even appreciate patterns of behavior without engaging with them. You can allow them to exist without inviting them in.

By simply not tuning in to or engaging with familiar patterns, or even by just engaging less, you can create the necessary space for new patterns to emerge.

Document your progress!

One way to help overcome this self-defeating habit is to collect evidence of your progress and successes. Keep a journal--specifically, a special journal of your personal successes and triumphs. I'm a big fan of different types of journals for different things.

If journaling is not your thing, keep a cookie jar or a little black book or a digital notepad or folder of voice-clips or a portfolio of sketches, and make a note or a mark or a symbolic reminder of your successes whenever you notice them. Whatever works for you is perfect.

Cultivate this habit and you will build momentum. Then, on the occasions you are feeling down, review some of them and help remind yourself of how far you have come, of the trials and struggles you have lived through and overcome. This can help you get back on track more quickly when you fall off.

While it's important to process negative emotions, limiting beliefs, fears, and resentments, it's equally necessary to develop the skill of seeing and celebrating your successes and wins. Like any habit, this takes practice.

Don't beat yourself up if it seems difficult at first. Simply return to your resolve to love yourself, improve, and make positive progress. Let go of self-defeating self-talk whenever you recognize it.

Build evidence in your favor. One way we self-sabotage is by not being honest with ourselves. Another is by allowing incongruent or self-defeating beliefs to govern our actions and decisions.

If you've been practicing the same patterns for a long time--years, decades, or perhaps lifetimes--you may unconsciously collect evidence to support a belief that you are defective or broken. Be patient with yourself and give yourself some grace.

The Shift. Own your emotions; Own your life.

The more you practice this, the more convincing the evidence becomes. The same is true when we collect evidence of our success. Focus on creating and collecting evidence of your successes and strengths instead of your failures and weaknesses.

Make a practice of collecting this evidence for yourself to help light your way out of despair. Keep a celebration journal, a scrapbook, or a 'cookie jar' of wins. Collect evidence of those positive moments and the things you've set out to do and accomplished. Over time, you can build a great 'arsenal' of evidence to help pull you up.

Believe in yourself!

She who believes she can, and she who believes she cannot, are both right.

Belief is a keystone of accomplishment, and it's an area where many humans fail before they even start. If you tell yourself you can't, then you probably won't.

A first step in this shift is to stop telling yourself you can't and at least believe there's a possibility. Maybe you can.

You can try adding the simple word "yet" to self-limiting stories that begin with "I can't" or "I don't" and see how it opens new possibilities in your story. Shift "I can't" to "I haven't yet", or "I don't know how" to "I haven't learned yet". While you are making this shift, try out the phrase "I think I can" as much as possible.

INVITATION TO ACTION: I invite you to take a few minutes to jot down any regular self-limiting

The Shift. Own your emotions; Own your life.

thoughts you catch yourself thinking often, and also to
begin to notice them as you go through your day, and
practice adding "yet" or "so far" to as many as you can.
Then tag on "I think I can…", "I wonder if…" or "Maybe I
can…". Play with possibility. Add a little space around
those statements where you feel there is none. You can do
it.

Here are a few of my personal favorites to get you started:

"I don't feel loveable…yet."

"I don't know how to do this…so far."

"I am not brave enough…yet."

Now you try.

We used to believe that running a mile in less than four
minutes was physically impossible. Then someone did it, it
got written into our history, and now many people know
they can do it.

We used to believe flight was impossible. Now we have
planes flying around the world every day and even send
rockets into space. Many things seem impossible until we
do them.

Believe that you can change your mindset and learn to stop
self-sabotaging. Believe that you can cultivate a life you
love. Believe that you are worthy of your own love. You'll
be closer to achieving this once you believe in your ability.
If you don't quite believe it yet, try to pretend that you do,
just for now.

The Shift. Own your emotions; Own your life.

You Are Having a Biological Experience

Remember, you don't procrastinate because you're lazy. You procrastinate because your brain chemistry isn't in sync with your intentions. When we're dysregulated-- overwhelmed, scattered, numb, or shut down--it's often a sign our neurochemicals need a quick reboot.

Understanding these five core neurochemicals can help you work with your brain and body--not against them-- especially when you feel stuck, overwhelmed, or out of sync.

Dopamine: *Drives motivation, anticipation, and goal pursuit.*
Dopamine helps you feel energized to take action and make progress toward your goals. When out of balance, it can lead to procrastination, boredom, distraction, or chasing quick dopamine hits (like sugar, scrolling, or starting new things without finishing).

To Re-regulate:

- Break tasks into small wins
- Check things off a list
- Add novelty or a mini-reward
- Visualize the reward and reconnect with your *why*

Norepinephrine: *Supports alertness, attention, and mental clarity.* It helps you engage with challenges, stay focused, and mentally "show up." When out of balance, you might feel foggy, anxious, restless, or freeze up when trying to start something.

To Re-regulate:

- Move your body (shake, jump, stretch)
- Splash cold water or use peppermint
- Use a timer or countdown to create urgency
- Get sunlight or fresh air

Cortisol: *Manages your stress response and keeps you responsive under pressure.* In balance, it gives you energy and resilience in tough situations. When dysregulated (especially too high for too long), it can cause tension, irritability, perfectionism, and eventual emotional or physical burnout.

To Re-regulate:

- Take long, slow exhales
- Reframe the pressure: "This is a draft, not a test"
- Ground yourself with your senses
- Gently stretch, sway, or walk

Oxytocin: *Creates feelings of safety, connection, and trust.* It's essential for emotional bonding and co-regulation with others. When low, you may feel isolated, numb, or unable to ask for help, even when you deeply want support.

To Re-regulate:

- Hug someone (or yourself)

The Shift. Own your emotions; Own your life.

- Spend time with a pet
- Text or talk to someone who feels safe
- Use loving self-talk or mirror work

Endorphins: *Provide natural pain relief and boost joy or lightness.* They help you bounce back from stress and feel more emotionally buoyant. When depleted, life can feel heavier, flatter, or emotionally dull—sometimes leading to unhealthy coping just to feel something.

To Re-regulate:

- Laugh, sing, dance, or move playfully
- Watch something funny
- Stretch and yawn
- Do something creative, silly, or expressive

Remember: You don't need to fix everything at once. One breath, one stretch, or one smile can begin to shift your chemistry. You're not lazy or broken--sometimes you're just low on the right fuel.

The tools in this book work because they shift these chemicals. You'll feel it when you:

Shake → norepinephrine spikes = energy returns
Hug or hum → oxytocin rises = safety returns
Sing, sway, or smile → endorphins flow = lightness returns
Breathe, pause, reframe → cortisol softens = clarity returns
Complete one tiny task → dopamine flows = motivation returns

The Shift. Own your emotions; Own your life.

You're not broken, but you could be working against your own chemistry. Regulation is the art of tuning your system gently, not forcing it to perform.

How can we stop the self-sabotage?

It is important to realize that self-sabotage is normal. Even the most successful humans self-sabotage sometimes. The trick is to learn to recognize when you are doing it, especially when it is particularly harmful to living the life you want and becoming the person you want to be.

Be willing to stand out, go alone, and hold yourself in a higher state, even when those around you do not. Be willing to be uncomfortable as you try new things and develop new skills.

Like most things, you can improve this with practice.

Many humans tend to stay in the lower states of consciousness, repeating the same self-defeating patterns. This is not because they are stupid or want to suffer, but because it's familiar and that's where the majority operate.

It's common to try to reduce ourselves to try to fit into the current 'over-culture' rather than cultivate our sense of true belonging to life or 'civilization' on a grander scale.

It's also common to use the idea of intimacy and love to manipulate and devastate one another. "Hurt people hurt people" as the saying goes.

Many of us have experienced trauma and betrayal of trust early in life and this can leave us feeling calloused or guarded to such an extent that we end up perpetuating the same wounds in others, often in those closest to us like our children and our partners.

Wounded people often lash out and try to hurt others. This can be seen as unconsciousness and incoherence. Try not to take it personally, because if you do, you might become incoherent and less conscious too.

Food for Thought: When I notice someone lashing out or hurting others intentionally, I imagine they're like a wounded animal tied to a post.

I realize they probably feel trapped in their own story of limitation and fear. I try to remember that this fear ultimately comes from an underinformed or underdeveloped sense of love or an unmet desire. This helps me not to take it personally. I can try to help and also keep myself safe.

Remember that when a person is wounded, they're not acting completely consciously. They aren't behaving rationally. While they might not intentionally hurt others, they're still likely to.

This is why it's important to treat angry or wounded people with compassion and not get too entangled with them or take their anger personally or internalize it and make it part of our own story, thereby perpetuating this downward spiraling cycle.

As soon as you accept full responsibility for your life, you might feel overwhelmed by all the mistakes you've made up to this point. You might feel guilty or ashamed for hurting others who tried to get close to you.

You might start wondering, "What even is the point?"

You might wallow in disbelief for a time, proclaiming, "This is not my beautiful life."

You might be tempted to slip back into that victim or limited mindset and get in your own way some more, continuing to play the "look what you made me do" game.

The Shift. Own your emotions; Own your life.

If you do, remember this is a normal part of the human condition.

Don't keep making the same mistake just because you've spent a lot of time making it. Remember, you can shift. Do your best to let go of the negative self-talk and focus on the values you want to cultivate in your life.

It's a very common human habit to blame others and slip into that victim mindset, looking at what's happening as if it's happening "to you."

It's up to you to 'take the wheel' of your own life, be the captain of your own ship, and drive your life forward in the direction you want it to go. With practice you can train your mind into better patterns of thought and become the master of your own destiny.

It's always tempting to blame it all on someone else and not take responsibility for our own mistakes or shortcomings. Sometimes it seems easier to give in to old patterns of blame, criticism, and resentment rather than set about cleaning up the messes we've made. It can be difficult to muster the courage to 'do your best to do better,' especially knowing you're likely to 'fail' again.

Please note I am NOT saying that everything is your fault and no one else ever victimized you. I am just saying it will not help you improve your life if you keep telling that story or focusing on that. Even if it is true, and perhaps even especially if it is true, it is important to realize you can learn to control what you give your attention to.

Society at large tends to fall to the lowest common denominator. If you don't first bring yourself to a higher frequency and learn to hold yourself there, it will be difficult to 'tap into' this higher frequency. However, if you do, you can then connect to other humans who are also 'tapping in,' and together, we can do incredible things. It's a dance of sorts; between holding yourself accountable to your values and learning to get 'in flow' with the collective of conscious beings.

I urge you to do it anyway, especially when it seems difficult. The alternative is to spiral further down into your own self-made hell. You are likely to drag many others down with you, even when you don't mean to. We all need each other to pull up, lift ourselves from our own despair, and focus on staying conscious and getting healthy so we can best face the coming storms.

In the same way that regular physical exercise develops a healthier body, regular mental practices develop a healthier mind. Learning to process your emotions in healthier ways will help you develop better emotional fitness. It takes time, and some days it will be easier than others. This is the dynamic dance of life.

Society at large will encourage you to slip back into mediocrity and disempowerment. As they say, "misery loves company," and people love to see others succeed-- until those others are succeeding more than they perceive themselves to be. At that point, they often turn a bit nasty.

The analogy of crabs in a crab pot is popular in this context. However, crabs don't pull each other back down in the pot because they don't want to see other crabs' escape. They pull each other down because they want to escape and will use any means they can, including grabbing other crabs, to try to pull themselves out.

Crabs in a crab pot are essentially wounded animals. Feeling trapped and overcome with a sense of impending doom, uncertain of what the future holds, they become relentlessly focused on escaping at any cost. Humans can be like this too.

However, we humans can also collaborate. We can learn and communicate when we rise above our fears and self-regulate our energetic state. We can work together in ways that crabs cannot.

While we do sometimes pull each other down out of envy, it's more often because we feel isolated, alone, and trapped. Sometimes, we unconsciously pull others down as we try to lift ourselves out of our own lower states.

The secret, then, is to elevate our own emotional and physical state from the inside. The key is to learn to communicate and cooperate more effectively with each other and with our own bodies, through our emotions.

We can cultivate more conscious coherence by deliberately elevating our energetic state and connecting to a broader field of consciousness.

Some people call this God. I like to think of it in terms of frequencies and coherence. Really, though, at least from my perspective, it's all the same stuff. This doesn't have to be metaphysical, but it can be.

Get to higher ground. Shift your perspective. Realize you are not alone.

There is much more to this Universe than a single human can fathom. When we connect our energy to other humans and raise our own vibration, we can do incredible things. This is what has allowed us to become so successful in life, and what can allow any single human to create more successful outcomes.

The Shift. Own your emotions; Own your life.

Set yourself up for success by taking a good hard look at your internal and external environments and seeing where you can make small adjustments that will have big positive effects.

Keep in mind, there are other humans who are also working to be in this higher, energetic flow state more of the time. I think it is exciting to consider that we might be in a collective shift towards a higher energetic state.

It's important not to fall into 'the pit of despair,' start 'playing the blame game,' or wallow in self-pity at this stage. Recognize that this is a natural part of the process and nothing to make a big deal about. Keep it in perspective.

It's an important step to begin recognizing when you are repeating self-defeating thoughts or actions. When you recognize an underlying belief that doesn't serve you in your quest to move closer to your personal goals and mission, appreciate that you've become more self-aware. Don't beat yourself up about it. Congratulate yourself for being self-aware. Then, shift.

If you do fall back into the pit of despair, realize this is still just a normal part of the process. You can make the Shift and change direction at any time.

It can be difficult to see evidence of progress at first. If you've been collecting evidence of your victimhood for a long time, it will likely take persistence to begin seeing the glimmers and sparks that show you are making progress.

If all this seems like too much right now, take heart, brave heart. You don't need to 'swallow the whole thing right now.' Just bite off a little bit. Take a tiny step in a better direction.

The Shift. Own your emotions; Own your life.

We've all been in that surreal, disheartened place of bewilderment and disappointment. We all know that feeling of failure, where we can clearly see that we caused our own hardship and sometimes hardship for others as well.

"I do not use other people's choices to hurt my own feelings." ~James-Olivia Chu Hillman

Understanding and Overcoming Self-Sabotage

Self-sabotage is a universal human experience. We all have moments where, despite wanting success or happiness, we find ourselves getting in our own way-- whether through procrastination, fear of failure, or negative self-talk.

The good news is, while self-sabotage is a natural tendency, we can learn to recognize it and train ourselves to overcome it. Research shows that with the right tools and awareness we can break free from these patterns and shift towards greater self-mastery.

A key reason why self-sabotage happens is due to a conflict between conscious goals and subconscious fears or limiting beliefs.

Research published in Personality and Social Psychology Bulletin found that self-sabotaging behavior often stems from self-protective mechanisms, where we subconsciously avoid taking risks because of fear--fear of failure, rejection, or even success.

While these behaviors may provide short-term relief, they ultimately hold us back from achieving our goals. The good news is that by bringing awareness to these patterns, we can start to dismantle them.

One effective way to overcome self-sabotage is through cognitive-behavioral techniques (CBT), which focus on identifying and changing the negative thought patterns that fuel self-sabotaging behaviors.

A study published in Behavior Research and Therapy showed that individuals who practiced cognitive restructuring--the process of challenging and reframing negative thoughts--were able to reduce self-sabotaging behaviors and improve overall performance. By consistently applying these techniques, we can rewire our thought patterns to support rather than hinder our progress.

It's important to recognize that none of these methodologies is failproof, and finding someone to work with can be challenging. My focus in this book is on methods that anyone can use for free, but there are many specialty methods that are worth looking into if you feel drawn to them and have the means.

Self-sabotage is also closely tied to self-worth and imposter syndrome, which are common underlying causes. Most people experience imposter syndrome at some point in their lives, where they feel undeserving of their accomplishments or fear being exposed as a fraud.

This internal conflict can lead to behaviors that undermine our efforts, as we struggle to reconcile our desire for success with our deep-seated fear of failure. Learning to challenge these beliefs is a crucial part of overcoming self-sabotage.

Additionally, neuroscience research shows that habits of self-sabotage are often linked to automatic brain responses--when we repeatedly engage in self-sabotaging behaviors, we create neural pathways that make these behaviors more ingrained. However, with neuroplasticity, the brain's ability to change and form new connections, we can rewire these pathways.

Through consistent practice of new, positive behaviors, we can effectively override old patterns and create new habits that support our goals.

The Shift. Own your emotions; Own your life.

The key to overcoming self-sabotage is training ourselves to recognize it and using tools like cognitive reframing, mindfulness, and self-compassion to break the cycle. Over time, with practice, we can transform our patterns of self-sabotage into self-support, giving ourselves the freedom to succeed on our own terms.

It is also important to do whatever you can to create internal and external support systems. Take care of your basic needs. Surround yourself with signals and signs that inspire you to take positive actions. Start to remove or clean up signals, signs, and relationships that drag you down.

Right now, even if you're feeling uncertain about how to proceed, celebrate yourself for coming this far and getting to this stage. Get in the habit of celebrating your successes, starting now.

Now that you're recognizing that you are the biggest thing getting in your own way, you can get to the important business of coming back into alignment with your truest, most authentic, uniquely-qualified-to-be-you self.

Though you might be thinking you can't possibly make it to where you want to go from where you are now, I assure you, that is simply your self-limiting default mode network talking. That's what your brain naturally thinks when it doesn't know something.

The brain's natural default is to look for the worst-case scenario, spot potential dangers, and keep you alive at any cost. It is simply trying to protect you. However, too much safety leads to the death of everything.

The Shift. Own your emotions; Own your life.

The Shift holds the keys to help you reprogram your default mode network and reticular activating system to serve you better.

You can change. In fact, change is inevitable. The question is, how much agency will you claim over the changes in your life?

Will you take the reins and steer yourself towards the goals you choose, or will you allow yourself to be blown around by the winds of change without taking up your own power of responsibility? The choice is always yours.

There are paths and shortcuts you don't know about yet. As you learn to trust yourself in this process of becoming, you will find the necessary clarity and skills becoming clearer as you get closer to them. You don't need to see the entire journey clearly to take the first step. You have already taken a big step by opening this book and coming this far.

If your mind insists on replaying your limiting beliefs, see if you can get them to lighten up a little, or perhaps set them aside temporarily to explore some 'what ifs' and rekindle some sparks of possibility in your life.

So, at least for right now, let's set down that limiting belief. Press pause on it, and just set it aside for now. You can always come back to it and press play again if you decide it better serves you.

The default mode is always there, willing to sweep you back into your repeating patterns. But for now, let's agree to set a goal to try out new tools and see if any of them lead to improvement. Deal? What have you got to lose?

The Shift. Own your emotions; Own your life.

Give Yourself a Gold Star!

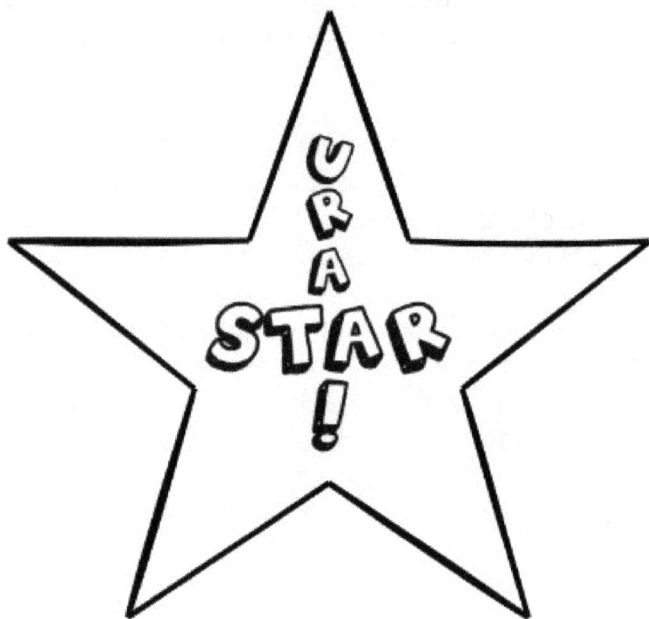

The Ant and the Elephant's Journey

Towards A Better Life:

Not very long ago, deep in the heart of the savanna, an ant found itself perched upon the back of an enormous elephant. The ant was determined to reach a distant valley--The Land of Milk and Honey"--where food and abundance were said to flow endlessly.

With its tiny legs and quick mind, the ant plotted a precise and efficient route to the valley. It shouted directions into the wind, convinced it could control the path forward.

"Faster! We must get there soon!" the ant would say. "Turn left here! ...Right now! ...This is the quickest way."

The elephant, however, lumbered and strolled slowly and with great purpose, stepping carefully and taking a path that the ant couldn't understand.

The ant grew frustrated and impatient, constantly scurrying around on the elephant's back, convinced that its tiny perspective was the only one that mattered.

Some days into their journey, as they approached a steep canyon, the ant saw a narrow bridge and urged the elephant to cross it. "This is the fastest way! We'll lose time if we don't take this route!"

But the elephant, sensing the fragility of the bridge relative to its own weight, and knowing of several other dangers that lay ahead, refused to move toward it. The elephant took a longer, winding path through the canyon floor.

The Shift. Own your emotions; Own your life.

The ant was furious. "You're too slow! You don't see the way I do. We'll never make it to the valley!"

Eventually, as the days passed, the ant began to notice that the elephant moved with a wisdom that the ant hadn't yet grasped. Where the ant saw only a straight line to the goal, the elephant saw the bigger picture—the hidden dangers, the natural rhythms of the land, and the need for balance, water, shelter, and rest.

As they journeyed on, the ant began to quiet its constant demands, learning to observe and trust the elephant's deeper instincts. It realized that although it could plan and strategize, the elephant had access to a higher view, one that connected to the subconscious flow of life, the rhythms of nature, and the unseen forces guiding their path.

Finally, they reached the valley—arriving not just safely, but at exactly the right time, when the rains had just come, and the valley was bursting with abundance. The ant marveled at how the journey had unfolded, recognizing that its conscious planning was valuable, but that it also needed the elephant's broader, intuitive wisdom to guide them to the right place, at the right moment.

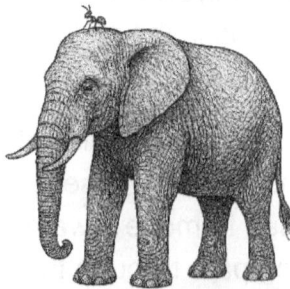

Colder-Warmer

Did you ever play the "hot-cold" hide-and-seek game? When you're searching for something, and someone tells you whether you're "getting warmer" or "getting colder," or "very hot" or "very cold"?

This is similar to how our limbic systems operate. We are either moving towards what our system thinks it wants to maintain homeostasis, or away from what it thinks it wants.

I find it helpful to think of my body's communication system as an infant or very young child. It is pure and simple in its desires, needs, and communication style. Your guidance system will tell you when you're out of alignment, off course, and not acting in accordance with your internal values. Learn to listen to your own guidance system with the same gentle compassion you would offer a young child.

I often hear people say they've learned not to trust their emotions, or someone else's emotions. It's common to get advice not to make decisions based on feelings or emotions.

This is partially true but only partly true. It is definitely best not to make most decisions when you're in a dysregulated state. When emotions or feelings are very strong— extremely high or extremely low—we are usually dysregulated and probably not thinking straight.

I think we are at our best when we can use logic and emotions to inform our decisions. Either one without the other leads to suboptimal results.

Another reason we might have learned not to pay attention to our emotions is that our perception of the intensity of our feelings or emotions is often NOT directly proportional to

171

The Shift. Own your emotions; Own your life.

the intensity of the situation and our need to act. In fact, similar to dealing with a young child, you might be wise to be more concerned when things are quieter than when they are dramatic and loud. However, if you learn to notice and name your feelings, and take some time to figure out why you feel the way you do, you'll discover that your feelings and emotions can offer great wisdom and guidance.

When you realize that your emotions are your body's way of communicating with you and that your emotions and your body are 'on your side', you might to see more clearly how becoming dysregulated distorts your ability to make healthy informed choices or communicate your needs and desires to others effectively.

You can begin to take responsibility for your own state of consciousness and elevate yourself or take a break to recover when you find you don't have the capacity to re-regulate. When you notice negative, self-defeating patterns, you can change them and improve your skills.

By doing this work on yourself, you can also help humanity move in the direction of more sanity, communication, and cooperation, rather than adding your personal energy to the chaos and dysfunction.

Learn to recognize that overwhelm is a signal from your system that you need to change your thoughts and actions.

IF YOU FIND YOURSELF IN THE PIT OF DESPAIR, STOP DIGGING, FIND THE STAIRS, OR DRAW A THIRD DOOR.

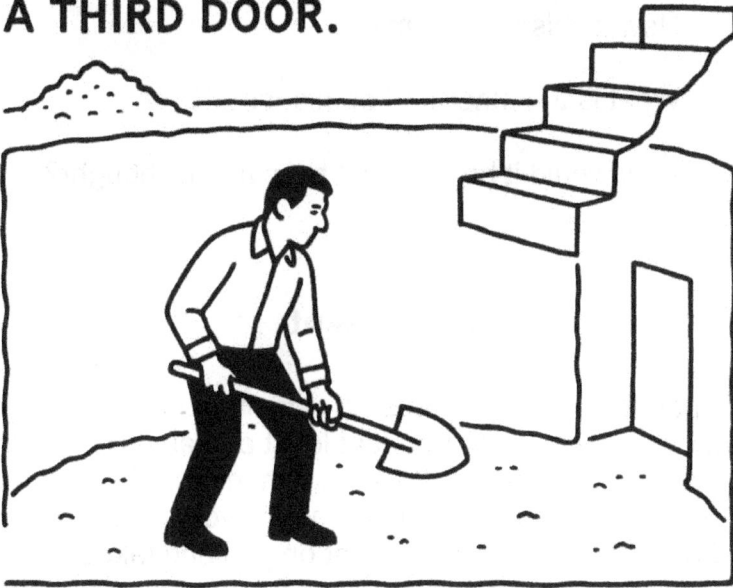

At least for a little while, just for a moment, right now—suspend disbelief and belief, open the doors to possibility. What have you got to lose?

Whenever and wherever you can, plant seeds of hope.

If you feel like you're "in too deep" in the "pit of despair" and don't believe there's a way out, take heart. Hope can exist if you choose to make space for it to sprout, take hold, and if you decide to cultivate it in your own heart. This is how humanity builds and passes on hope--from generation to

The Shift. Own your emotions; Own your life.

generation, from relationship to relationship, from story to story.

You can pull yourself out of the pit very easily when you start to ask and answer these questions honestly:

How is this serving me?

What is the other end of this "stick"?

How would it be if I didn't believe this thought?

Your Elephant and Your Ant

Let's pause here and address an elephant in the room. You are most likely thinking about at least one aspect of your life that feels hopeless to change right now. Perhaps you lost your legs in an accident, or maybe you are caring for a child or parent who is dependent on you and takes so much of your energy that you can't fathom how it will ever be okay.

Put a small layer of possibility around that thought for now. Remember, things can always be worse, and they can always get better.

If you can't find a way to feel okay about it, try to leave it alone for the time being. Just do the best you can from where you are right now. It will get easier with practice.

I am not asking you to believe in the impossible. I am simply asking you to "suspend your disbelief" for a time, similar to how you might when watching a movie.

The Shift. Own your emotions; Own your life.

Imagine what it might be like if you could get around that impossible obstacle and allow yourself to contemplate the possibilities of your life outside the confines of your limitations, even if just for a short time. Imagine what that would FEEL like.

I am also not saying you didn't get delt a shitty hand in life. I don't know if you did or did not. I do know that you can play a good hand poorly and a bad hand well.

I hope you will choose to play whatever circumstances life deals you to the best of your ability and feel good about it.

Throughout human history, people have documented their journeys through these "dark nights of the soul." We need each other as much as ever right now. Your successful shift matters. You matter.

We all serve as examples or warnings to others along the way. It is up to you to determine and cultivate how much of your story will be a positive signpost. What will be good examples for others, and what will be warnings? This will get easier with practice.

In business, you hear the saying: "You are the sum of the five people you spend the most time around (or thinking about)" and this is true in many ways. This is another good reason to be selective about who you spend your time with.

Your friends, business associates, intimate partners, and also your enemies, or the ideas you choose to push against, have an impact on your life. It's important to choose your friends and your enemies wisely. Think about the people you spend time around or thinking about, carefully.

The Shift. Own your emotions; Own your life.

There are parts of this journey where you will find much-needed support. However, the hardest parts of this journey are those you can only do alone. I don't mean to downplay how it feels though. Sometimes, it feels like the sky is falling and it's the end of the world.

This is your invitation to step out of that story for just a moment. Suspend that belief, that way of thinking, just temporarily.

Consider that, just like in the story of Chicken Little, the sky that appears to be falling could be a misinterpretation of something far less catastrophic, like a falling leaf.

Is it possible that the sky isn't actually falling?

If it is falling, does screaming, crying, or melting down into a feeble puddle help at all? Not usually.

Can you see that history gives us evidence that things go on more often than not?

Can we agree that everything is ultimately temporary, at least on a long enough timeline?

Can you imagine entertaining the idea that it might be possible to untangle all those knots and feel clear and coherent again?

Remember, you've made it this far; no doubt you've successfully navigated a lot of this terrain before. You are stronger than you think.

Check-in with your body and remember that humans have been enduring struggles and triumphs for thousands of years. In fact, all of our greatest achievements have come from overcoming great challenges.

The Shift. Own your emotions; Own your life.

See if you can create a small space of possibility for yourself to heal. Give yourself permission to take a little more time to figure this out.

Take all the time you need, but also, start now.

Find the keys to unlock your unique gifts, which are always gems hidden in our unique shadows.

See if you can shift your perception and your energy a little bit. That is all it takes to build upon--one tiny spark of hope.

Do not lose heart! Remember that struggle is a normal part of the process. It is not as bad as you think. It is probably both worse and better than you think.

The Ant on the Back of the Elephant in the Room

Your subconscious is vastly more influential to your behaviors and beliefs than your consciousness. You might see the relationship between the conscious and subconscious depicted as an iceberg, where 90% of it is below the surface and the 10% you can see represents your consciousness--what you are aware of.

The ratio is probably closer to 99.999% subconscious and superconscious, and 0.0001% conscious--closer to the ratio of an elephant to an ant.

Your subconscious (and our collective super-consciousness) is vast in comparison to what you are consciously aware of at any point. Your body is comprised of an estimated 30–80 trillion cells (depending on how we

177

The Shift. Own your emotions; Own your life.

imagine counting them), which are constantly taking in and exchanging data.

Our bodies are interacting with our internal and external environments and communicating in ways we haven't even thought of yet. There is a whole lot more going on under the surface than we can figure out with our conscious minds. This is why paying attention to your energetic state and learning to cultivate coherence in your body is so valuable.

Your subconscious is more like an elephant compared to your conscious "ant" mind. I liken it to a tiny sugar ant walking on an elephant's back. That little ant is going to get a lot farther a lot faster if it's going in the same direction as the elephant.

We often consciously strive towards our goals while the elephant of our subconsciousness is lumbering along in a completely different direction. This is why it is important to spend time getting to "know thyself," and why talk therapy and various ways of remembering our past and unveiling our deeper, underlying beliefs can be helpful. It helps us untangle and understand the ways we are self-sabotaging. We are highly influenced by how well these two aspects of ourselves are aligned.

Coherence in your body is a signal that the ant of your conscious mind and the elephant of your subconscious are moving in the same, or at least more congruent, directions. It's the equivalent of "getting warmer" in that childhood game.

Dysregulation or incongruence is a signal that your ant and your elephant are not moving in the same direction. This is like your body saying, "you are getting colder."

The Shift. Own your emotions; Own your life.

Regaining coherence, alignment, or integrity between your subconscious programming and your conscious desires should become your first priority. When this doesn't feel possible, do the best you can, and try to remember that this is still a success--especially compared to the alternative. If you try and fail, congratulate yourself for trying, and try again.

Your subconscious includes stored memories and knowledge you can recall but aren't thinking about all the time and also things you are unconscious of but are influencing your decisions, like your repressed memories and suppressed feelings.

The superconscious includes generational, genetic information inherited from your ancestors and previous generations, as well as the time in human history, the cultures, and families you are born into.

The superconscious, the subconscious, and the infinitely vast void make up your unconsciousness. All that translates to information, or data, that you are receiving and not necessarily aware of until you get a feeling.

A better analogy might be a dancing bundle of crystallized light on a speck of dust, hurtling through a cosmos of space so vast we cannot perceive any end to it.

On some level, depending on the scope of the lens you look at us through, we are tiny, shiny specks of something far more vast than our conscious minds can comprehend. There is much more going on in and around you than you are aware of.

We repeat the same patterns in an unconscious attempt to create different results. By becoming aware of the underlying beliefs that cause us to create and recreate these patterns, we can consciously change them. When we realize they no longer serve us and maybe getting in the way of us becoming the person we want to be, we are making progress toward positive changes. We are getting warmer.

This is why many people use prayer or meditation. I don't believe it absolutely has to be one of these tried-and-true ways, but I do recommend you find a practice that works for you to regularly check in with your energetic state. Develop a practice of re-tuning yourself to the greater frequencies of life beginning with the frequencies of your own body.

Remember, there isn't just 'one way' to do this, although there are many ways others have explored that you can learn from. If you are unclear about where to start, 'imitate a master' until you begin to develop your own way. Then, when you are more comfortable and/or have hopefully developed some healthy strategies and habits, make sure you are doing things your own unique way--the way that is most authentic to you.

Using Your Feelings as a Guidance System…

"Warm, warmer, hot, colder, cold…"

Think of that uneasy feeling, that feeling of disorder and dysfunction, as a misalignment between your ant and your elephant. As your ant moves more and more against the direction of your values, the distortions and dysfunction will grow stronger and stronger. This is your body telling you to "turn"! Adjust your course! "You are getting colder!" Take heed. Listen to your heart. Your body knows the way instinctively, and your conscious input will help influence your own instincts.

If you simply suppress your feelings or armor yourself against the feelings of being off course, you can end up far removed from your true nature. Your natural state is to be coherent. Your whole self wants to be in integrity. All you need to do is relax.

Take your foot off the gas when it feels like you might be going the wrong way. Stop resisting, fighting, and focusing on what is wrong in your life. You will naturally come back into alignment.

This is truer if you surround yourself with others who are also in coherence, and harder to do if you are surrounded by people who are stuck in the struggle. We humans are connected, and our energetic states are contagious to one another. This is why they say you are the combination of the five people you spend the most time with, and why it is important to choose your friends and colleagues wisely.

Of course, sometimes danger and the unknown are things we do want to get through. With practice, you will get better at bringing your awareness into your body to check for alignment and listen to your own intuition for guidance.

As you get more in touch with your underlying desires and bring more of your subconscious into the light of consciousness, you will gain congruence and alignment of your conscious actions with your subconscious needs and desires.

By its nature, the subconscious will always be much vaster than your conscious mind. This is why it is also important to utilize tools that address your energetic state overall. We can consciously participate in the unconscious programs that are running in the background, and we can improve the efficiency and effectiveness with which they are running.

Do you know what you know?

There are things you know, things you don't know, things you don't know you don't know, and things you don't know you know. This is the source of much of your self-sabotage--the things you don't know you know, but your body does.

We tend to think it is mostly the things we don't know we don't know that get in our way or knock us down, and indeed, sometimes what we think we know and do not can trip us up.

There is a lot of information our bodies are taking in all the time though, that we are mostly unaware of, and this is playing a huge role in our overall experience. This is largely the information we are prone to misinterpret if we have not taken the time to learn the language of our bodies chemical signals.

Very often, instead of developing any logical understanding or intuitive awareness, we default to shitty stories about ourselves or others.

When you start paying more attention to your energetic state and invite more of your subconscious to be illuminated, you'll begin to see how beautifully orchestrated everything is.

I'm not going to tell you that's evidence of anything because I'm not sure it is, but I can tell you that understanding this, in whatever way you can, will be a key to unlocking your stored capacity.

Pattern recognition and the pause

What are the patterns in your life showing you?

The patterns you begin to recognize in your own life can be the keys to unlocking insights into how the very things that are getting in your way can also be your greatest superpower.

Anytime you find yourself thinking, "Why does this always happen to me?" or feeling frustrated because you're caught in an episode of Groundhog Day, take a moment to congratulate yourself for recognizing that pattern, and pause.

Use a brief pause, a moment of awareness, to take note of what is going on around you and in your life.

Notice what is going on inside you--in your thoughts/mind and in your body--when you realize you're in a familiar, self-defeating, or limiting pattern.

If you don't know why you have a certain feeling or think maybe you don't want it anymore, get curious. Ask yourself, "How is this serving me?"

Chaos is simply 'that which is outside our ability to see the pattern of.' In a way, this is similar to what many humans call God. It may seem like the opposite end of it since most of us think of God as a 'divine order,' but really, this is just that we are not yet capable of seeing the order in it.

The Shift. Own your emotions; Own your life.

To my perception, "God" is what we see as ordered but beyond our ability to fully comprehend. We often ascribe 'metaphysical' or magical properties to the aspects that feel 'good,' and chaos to the other end of the same stick.

Chaos is what we perceive as dark and disordered, but it is also that which is merely larger than our ability to see the order in. Things we once found chaotic invariably turn out to have a rhythm and a pattern when you 'zoom out' far enough in time and space. Exploding stars make perfect sense in the context of the dancing arms of galaxies.

"...by the time you are real, most of your hair has been loved off, and your eyes drop out and you get loose in the joints and very shabby. But these things don't matter at all, because once you are real you can't be ugly, except to people who don't understand." (The Velveteen Rabbit)

Looking forward and back

David Goggins is another remarkable person with a very inspiring life story (look into it if you're not familiar), and one of the tools he talks about using is a type of self-loathing to overcome his darkest moments. He explains a way to rise rather than fall to self-defeat is to think about how your whole life can change in a split second and cultivate extreme self-discipline. He has said he thinks back on the feeling he used to have of being a failure and uses that as fuel to push himself towards his goals in the present.

Tim Ferris, who also has a remarkable life story worth investigating, is best known for his Four-Hour Work-Week series. In that book he describes a process of looking forward and imagining the worst-case scenario in order to prepare, plan, and bolster yourself against the potential upsets that come from navigating the sometimes turbulent seas of life.

The Shift. Own your emotions; Own your life.

I like to imagine myself from the future, looking back at myself in the present. These are all useful techniques to help Shift your perspective and your emotional state.

Imagine looking back on the current moment from your last moment. By collapsing the timeline of your life, you can gain a sense of clarity and tap into a source of energy you might not know you have.

When you imagine yourself old and at the end of your life:

Who do you want to be?

What do you hope others say and think about you?

What might you regret if you don't at least try to become it?

What unique parts of you are dying right now, and

What are you willing to do to really discover, uncover, and cultivate the one, true, beautiful, you?

What is one thing you can do today that your future self will thank you for tomorrow?

How Understanding Our Beliefs Drives Change

In the context of self-sabotage, it's essential to recognize that the conscious mind--the "ant"--may have clear goals and desires, but it is often the subconscious mind--the "elephant"--that steers the journey.

The ant represents our conscious efforts, like setting goals or trying to build new habits, but the elephant, carrying our deeper beliefs, values, and fears, often holds more power over our decisions and behaviors.

If we don't understand what's driving the elephant, it can be nearly impossible to overcome patterns of self-sabotage.

The key is learning to align the conscious mind (the ant) with the subconscious (the elephant) so they can work together toward positive change.

Uncovering and understanding our subconscious beliefs plays a crucial role in breaking self-sabotaging patterns. A great deal of our behavior is influenced by subconscious beliefs we aren't even fully aware of.

These beliefs are often rooted in early experiences, conditioning, or unresolved emotional conflicts, and they can drive behaviors that contradict our conscious desires.

For example, if your subconscious belief is that "success will lead to rejection," even though you consciously want to succeed, your elephant may hold you back, and your tiny conscious ant might feel bewildered about why you can't seem to make any real progress.

By bringing these subconscious patterns to the surface, we can begin to ask better questions and transform them.

The Shift. Own your emotions; Own your life.

One powerful way to align the ant and the elephant is through mindfulness and reflective practices. A 2014 study found that mindfulness meditation significantly increased participants' awareness of their unconscious thought patterns, allowing them to recognize self-sabotaging behaviors and make more deliberate choices.

By creating time and space for reflection in our lives, we can become more attuned to the deeper beliefs that drive our actions and, importantly, begin to challenge and sometimes change them.

Cognitive dissonance theory, first introduced by Leon Festinger in the 1950s, also supports this approach. Cognitive dissonance occurs when there's a conflict between our conscious goals and our underlying beliefs, creating discomfort that can lead to self-sabotaging behavior.

A study published in the Personality and Social Psychology Bulletin found that people who resolved this dissonance by either adjusting their beliefs or aligning their behaviors experienced greater emotional clarity and goal fulfillment. This reinforces the idea that understanding and reshaping our beliefs can help us move in alignment with what we consciously want.

This means we must do the inner work of challenging old beliefs and installing new, empowering ones. Neuro-linguistic programming (NLP) is one method that helps people become aware of and reframe limiting beliefs. NLP techniques like 'belief change' and 'anchoring' enable individuals to replace negative, subconscious beliefs with new, positive associations.

Once these shifts happen on the level of your subconscious 'elephant', your conscious 'ant' can guide

The Shift. Own your emotions; Own your life.

you toward your goals with much more ease, without constant internal friction.

The lesson here is that change doesn't only come from willpower or conscious effort (the ant). True, lasting change comes from addressing the deeper, often hidden, beliefs that steer the elephant.

By understanding what's driving us beneath the surface, we can harness the power of the elephant and move forward with a sense of flow, rather than resistance.

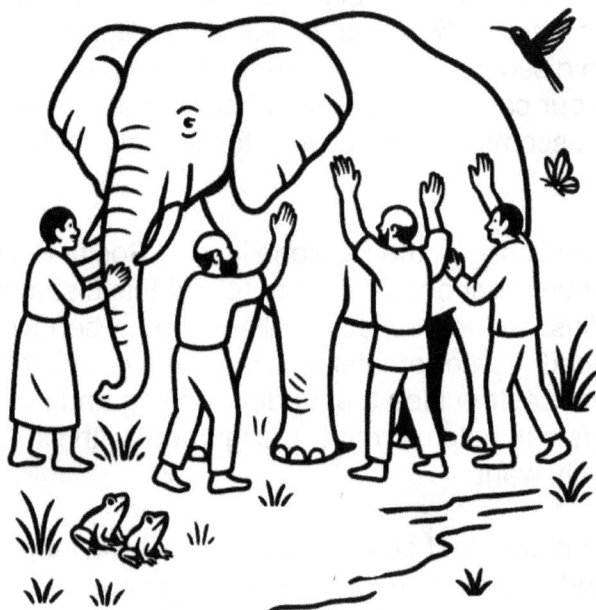

Five Blind Men and the Elephant

Once, in a different time, in a village far away, there lived five blind men. One day, the villagers excitedly told them that a grand elephant had arrived in the town square. Although the blind men had never encountered an elephant before, their curiosity was piqued. They decided to visit the elephant and learn more about this magnificent creature for themselves.

When they reached the elephant, each man approached a different part of the animal, eager to understand what an elephant was like.

The first blind man, feeling the elephant's leg, declared, "Ah! An elephant is strong and solid, like a tree trunk. It stands tall and firm, rooted in the earth."

The second man, who had grasped the elephant's tusk, disagreed. "No, no, you're mistaken! An elephant is sharp and smooth, like a spear."

The third blind man, with his hands on the elephant's side, shook his head. "You're both wrong. The elephant is broad and flat like a wall. It's sturdy and immovable."

The fourth man, who had grabbed the elephant's ear, laughed and said, "Not at all! This elephant is thin and flexible, like a fan. It's light and moves with the breeze."

Finally, the fifth blind man, holding onto the elephant's tail, concluded, "No, my friends, you're all wrong. The elephant is long and thin like a rope."

189

The Shift. Own your emotions; Own your life.

The five blind men began to argue, each absolutely certain that his experience of the elephant was the correct one.

"You must be mistaken!" they each said to one another. "I know what an elephant is really like!"

As their voices rose in frustration, a wise old man approached them and said, "You are all right, and yet none of you is completely right. Each of you has touched only a part of the elephant, and so each of you knows only a part of the truth. To understand the whole elephant, you must combine your experiences."

The blind men fell silent, realizing that their individual perceptions, though true to their own experiences, were incomplete. Only by considering each other's perspectives could they begin to understand the full reality of the elephant.

Just like the blind men and the elephant, we often only grasp parts of a larger truth. In life, each of us brings our own experiences, beliefs, and perspectives to the table, but these are just pieces of a more complex whole. Each person's journey is unique, and true mastery comes from integrating diverse perspectives, tools, and approaches.

Summary of Chapter Four:

Your emotions are not random, meaningless, or defects. They are also not 'facts.' They are signs and signals--clues you can use as guidance. Emotions, feelings, and intuitions are your body telling you when your elephant and your ant are, or are not, moving in the same direction. With practice, you can learn to develop a healthier relationship with your emotions, and this can improve your life significantly.

If you are living out of alignment with your underlying values, you will experience increasingly disruptive and distorted emotions as your body tries to guide you back into alignment. This includes, and begins with, your basic bodily functions.

We all need clean air, fresh water, nourishment, gentle touch and movement. We can survive, but it may be impossible to thrive without these basic needs met.

We all crave some security and some surprise. This is part of the dynamic dance of being alive.

Our current paradigm of labeling so many things as disorders can be harmful to our healing process. When we believe these are permanent states or defects rather than tools to help us steer our lives, we can miss the opportunities they hold.

I encourage you to question any narrative that tells you that you are defective, broken, incurable, or stuck where you are.

Distracting, drugging, or wallowing in our emotions instead of using them for fuel is an absurdity that I look forward to seeing us transcend.

The Shift. Own your emotions; Own your life.

I don't know anyone who hasn't experienced self-sabotage to some degree. If you're anything like me, you may be so familiar with it that sometimes it almost seems like a strange friend.

It could even be that you have developed an addiction to your own dysregulated chemistry. There are many reasons we self-sabotage and luckily, more than one way out. We can all become more emotionally fit with practice.

Current 'Western civilization' has normalized dysfunction and convinced people that living half-alive is the best we can hope for. This, my not-so-strange friend, is much more 'normal' than you might think. And yet, we can do much better. In fact, your resistance and self-sabotage can be a key to unlocking undiscovered and powerfully creative aspects of yourself.

This is your invitation to unlock a new level of your underdeveloped superpower. If you're willing to put down your judgments, shame, and blame, and get curious about why you feel the way you do, your resistance can become a clue, unique to you.

It Could Always Be Worse

There's an old Yiddish folktale about a poor man who lived with his wife, his six children, and his elderly mother in a tiny, cramped house. Life was hard, and everyone was always on top of each other, bickering and complaining. The man was at his wit's end, so he went to the wise rabbi for advice.

"Things are really bad, rabbi. I don't think they could be much worse." The man explained his woes to the rabbi.

The rabbi listened carefully and stroked his long white beard. "Tell me, good man, do you have any chickens?"

"Yes, rabbi. We are blessed with six hens and one young rooster."

"Excellent! Such a blessing!" the rabbi exclaimed. "You must go home at once and put the hens and the young rooster in the hut, and whatever you do, do not let them out."

The man was quite puzzled and even more distraught, but he did as the rabbi advised.

A week later, the man returned to the rabbi, more frustrated than before. "Rabbi," he said, "the house is even more crowded and noisy now with the chickens in it. My wife is as angry as the hens! It really couldn't be any worse! There are feathers in the soup! What should I do?"

The rabbi nodded thoughtfully and stroked his long, white beard. "I see. I see." He said. "Did you say you have a goat, dear man?"

The Shift. Own your emotions; Own your life.

"Yes, yes, Rabbi." We do have one goat." The man frowned and looked at the ground.

"Good, good." Said the rabbi. "Such a blessing! ...You must bring the goat into the hut as well then, and whatever you do, don't let it out!".

The man thought the rabbi might be losing his mind, but again he followed the advice.

A week later, the man came back to the rabbi, nearly at his breaking point. "Rabbi, it's unbearable! Things could not be worse! The house is complete chaos with the chickens, the goat, and all of us crowded together. My mother is angry from morning to night, rabbi. What do I do now?"

Again, the rabbi stroked his long white beard. He peered at the man and leaned forward. "Tell me, good man...do you have a cow?"

"Oh, no, rabbi. I mean, yes, we do have a cow but, please rabbi, we need some peace..."

"Good, Good. Such a blessing!" The rabbi smiled. "Go home, good man." The rabbi looked at him sternly with his piercing blue eyes. "Put the cow in the hut, and whatever you do, do not let her out."

The man walked home quite miserable and dragged his feet all the way home. His wife snarled and growled at him as he did as the rabbi had directed. Everyone in the hut had such a miserable week they were all finding new chores to do outside to keep themselves distracted. The following sabbath the man was eager to speak to the rabbi.

The Shift. Own your emotions; Own your life.

This time he spent several hours meditating outside before sunrise and then managed to enjoy a peaceful walk before he saw the rabbi.

"Good morning, rabbi. I really hope you have some fresh advice for me this week rabbi, because I really want my family to get along." The man smiled at the rabbi for the first time.

The rabbi looked back at him calmly and stroked his long white beard. Finally he said, "Good, good. Such a blessing... Now, go home and take the chickens and the goat and the cow back outside. Clean the hut and tell your wife to make a good supper for your family to enjoy together."

The man did as he was told. The next week, he returned to the rabbi with a big smile on his face. "Rabbi," he said, "the house is so quiet and spacious now! I can't believe how much room we had all along!"

The rabbi smiled and nodded and stroked his long white beard.

Sometimes we need to change our perspective to see how lucky we really are.

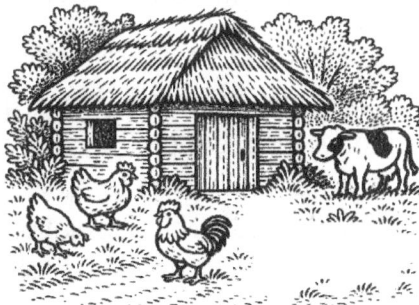

Real People Who Inspire Me:

Michael Jordan: The Ups and Downs of Struggling with One's Nature

Michael Jordan's career is often remembered as a flawless triumph, marked by championships, MVP awards, and game-winning shots. Under the surface, however, Jordan's story is one of intense struggle with the very beliefs and nature that made him great.

Throughout his life, he has faced personal and professional challenges that highlight how even the most successful people can wrestle with their internal stories and tendencies--sometimes to their advantage, and other times to their detriment.

Early in his basketball career, Michael Jordan faced a major setback when he was cut from his high school basketball team. At that moment, he had a choice: let the sting of rejection sabotage his potential, or use it as fuel to push harder. We all know what he chose.

Jordan went on to become the most iconic basketball player in history, known for his competitiveness, mental toughness, and willingness to outwork everyone else.

Jordan's infamous "win at all costs" mentality propelled him to six NBA championships and made him a global legend. Yet that same mindset also led to struggles in his personal life, and later in his career. His fiery temperament, gambling controversies, and strained relationships with teammates are well-documented, underscoring the double-edged nature of his drive.

David Choe: The Artist of Transformation

David Choe's life and work are a testament to the power of courage, creativity, and the willingness to embrace change. As an artist, storyteller, and cultural figure, he has inspired millions not only through his talent but through his raw vulnerability and relentless exploration of the human experience. His journey--marked by struggle, transformation, and cycles of reinvention--offers profound lessons from his own journey of self-mastery and struggles with emotional regulation.

David Choe's early years were defined by chaos and rebellion. Growing up in Los Angeles, he found refuge in graffiti, using art as a way to express the turmoil he felt inside. His bold, unapologetic style quickly gained attention, propelling him into the world of street art. However, his rise to fame was accompanied by battles with addiction, self-destructive behavior, and deep emotional struggles.

At one point, Choe faced a turning point after spending time in jail for shoplifting in Japan. This period of isolation forced him to confront his own shadow--the parts of himself that he had been running from. He began to see his art not just as a way to rebel but as a tool for self-reflection and healing.

Through his work, he explored themes of vulnerability, identity, and impermanence, translating his inner chaos onto canvas in ways that resonated deeply with others.

What makes David Choe truly inspiring is his courage to lay bare his flaws and struggles. He has spoken openly about his battles with depression, anxiety, and compulsive behaviors, creating a space for others to confront their own shadows. This willingness to be vulnerable is a recurring theme in his art and storytelling, demonstrating that strength comes not from hiding our pain but from facing it head-on.

Choe's journey of transformation became even more pronounced in recent years as he turned to tools like meditation, therapy, and breathwork to regulate his emotions and cultivate self-awareness. His exploration of mindfulness practices reflects his commitment to growth, showing that even amidst struggle, it is possible to find clarity and peace. These tools became anchors for him, helping him break free from cycles of self-sabotage and channel his energy into constructive, meaningful work.

Choe's story is about creative freedom and the courage to change. After achieving financial success, he could have coasted on his reputation, but he chose instead to delve deeper into his personal growth. He has continually reinvented himself, using his platform to discuss topics like emotional regulation, connection, and the value of self-expression.

Trevor Noah: Turning Pain into Humor and Connection

Trevor Noah's childhood was marked by the profound shadow of apartheid in South Africa. His best-selling book, Born a Crime, was highly influential for me in coming to a broader understanding of some of the dynamics of what we call "race". As a biracial child--born to a Black mother and a white father--Trevor's existence was considered illegal under the regime's oppressive laws.

Growing up, Trevor struggled with identity, belonging, and the systemic racism that permeated his world. Yet, instead of succumbing to bitterness, he learned to navigate these challenges with humor and curiosity.

Noah's ability to use humor as a tool for connection and healing reflects a deep integration of his shadow and is the thing I find most inspiring about him. He embraced the painful realities of his upbringing, turning them into stories that shed light on injustice while fostering empathy.

Born a Crime exemplifies how facing one's shadow--in this case, societal rejection and the pain of displacement—can lead to emotional resilience and a powerful sense of purpose.

By reframing his experiences, Trevor transformed his struggles into a platform for understanding and dialogue. His story teaches us that resilience often comes from leaning into our vulnerabilities, using them to build bridges rather than walls. He embodies the archetype of the Storyteller, whose voice inspires change and fosters connection.

INVITATION TO ACTION: I invite you to take out a notebook/your healing/work/shifting journal and reflect on the ways you self sabotage. A clue might be if the same pattern keeps happening over and over again.

The Shift. Own your emotions; Own your life.

In fact, whenever you find yourself thinking some version of "Why does this always happen to me?" it's a pretty safe bet that you are the common factor in a variety of scenarios. Jot down the first few that come to mind, and then ask yourself:

How is this serving me? Keep asking yourself the same question until you get to some new epiphany, or find yourself able to shift the story to something at least a little better.

For example: A common way I used to self-sabotage was by getting intimately entangled with unavailable men. With hindsight I could see clearly that the signs were all there that he was unavailable, yet I would still ignore them.

How was this serving me? I think I was trying to get love, feeding my ego by feeling desired...deeper than that, it has served a habitual pattern I have of feeling elated, then feeling shunned or scored or abandoned...it occurs to me I may have an addiction to feeling abandoned because this was a common pattern in my infancy and childhood...so it makes some sense that I do it to myself--self-abandon before someone else can abandon me...also I get energized (then exhausted) from what I call 'the push back'.

The Shift. Own your emotions; Own your life.

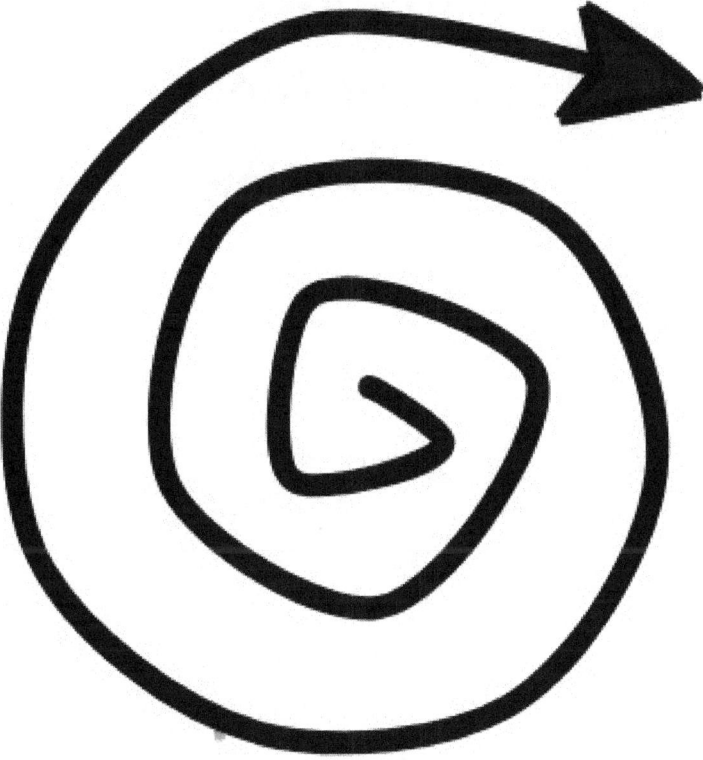

Part Two

Build Your Tool Kit

& Do the Work

CHAPTER 5

"NOT ONE WAY"

BUILD YOUR CUSTOM TOOLKIT FOR EMOTIONAL FITNESS

"The right tools limit mistakes." — Peter Sage

Let's dive into the work of building your custom toolkit for emotional fitness and personal mastery. It's important to remember that there isn't just 'one way' to do this correctly. These practices take time and patience, and while no single method is universally perfect, some basic principles tend to work for most people most of the time.

You don't need to completely reinvent the wheel, though you may need to put your unique spin on it. Some practices may come easily to you, while others might take more time. Some may be only partially effective, and some might not work for you at all.

The key to success is persistence. When you feel overwhelmed, pause and adjust. Breathe, and begin again. Find what works for you and let go of what doesn't.

Remember, the subconscious is vast compared to your conscious mind--think of the ant and the elephant analogy.

203

The Shift. Own your emotions; Own your life.

While you can make progress using your conscious mind, your progress can be much greater and faster if you tap into the power of your unconscious or subconscious mind. This is where art therapy, music, laughter, and what we often call metaphysical or supernatural practices can be highly effective.

I've done my best to compile and synthesize the resources and tools currently available, but I'm certain there are others I've missed, and new modalities will continue to emerge. As I've mentioned, and want to stress again, there isn't just one path to mastery. It's up to you to find and use what works best for you.

This chapter is an overview of tools and techniques I've found helpful, interesting, or currently popular. Remember, building your custom toolkit doesn't have to look like anyone else's. While many tools work well for most people, your toolkit should be tailored to your needs.

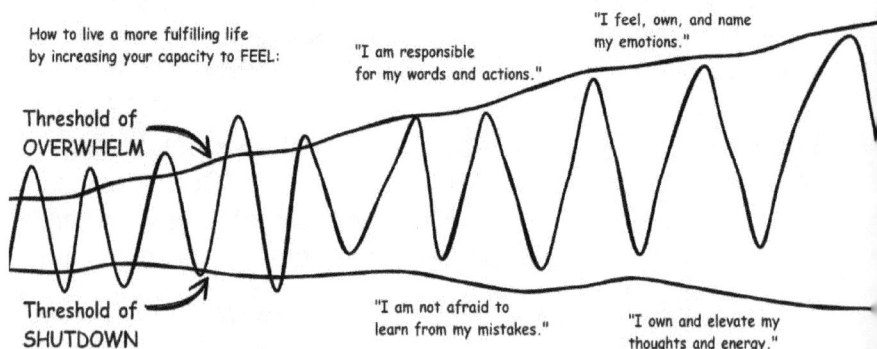

How to live a more fulfilling life by increasing your capacity to FEEL:

Threshold of OVERWHELM

Threshold of SHUTDOWN

"I am responsible for my words and actions."

"I feel, own, and name my emotions."

"I am not afraid to learn from my mistakes."

"I own and elevate my thoughts and energy."

The Fundamental Building Blocks

At the core of The Shift are simple yet powerful tools: pausing, questioning, breathing, moving, shifting awareness, relaxing, lightening up, and reframing. These foundational techniques are supported by research that demonstrates their ability to improve emotional regulation, increase self-mastery, and help us respond to life's challenges with intention rather than reaction. They are also free and readily available to nearly all of us, nearly all the time. Here's how each of these tools works, along with research backing their effectiveness.

Pausing

Pausing is often the first step in breaking automatic emotional reactions. By creating a gap between stimulus and response, we give ourselves the chance to reflect before acting. Research published in Frontiers in Psychology in 2014 shows that mindfulness practices, which emphasize pausing and becoming aware of the present moment, lead to greater emotional regulation and a reduction in impulsive behaviors. The study highlights that pausing allows the brain's prefrontal cortex—responsible for decision-making and self-control—to engage, overriding the amygdala's automatic fear or stress response.

Questioning

Questioning our thoughts and beliefs is crucial for rewiring emotional patterns. When we ask, "Is this true?" or "Is there another way to see this?", we engage in cognitive reappraisal. A study in the Journal of Neuroscience found that cognitive reappraisal, which involves questioning and reframing thoughts, significantly reduces emotional intensity by activating the dorsolateral prefrontal cortex, the brain area responsible for cognitive control. This process

The Shift. Own your emotions; Own your life.

helps us see situations in a more balanced way and make more conscious decisions.

Breathing

Controlled breathing is one of the most immediate ways to regulate the nervous system. To start with, just bring your attention to your breathing more often. See if you can slow it down, smooth it out, make it deeper and more regular.

There are several specific breathing exercises that can help regulate or reset your nervous system. A good place to start is to bring your awareness to your breath and start to make each breathe a bit slower and deeper if you can. Relax your shoulders, lengthen your spine, and expand your belly if you can.

Research shows that slow, deep breathing activates the parasympathetic nervous system and promotes relaxation. A study published in The Journal of Neurophysiology demonstrated that deep, diaphragmatic breathing lowers cortisol levels--the hormone associated with stress--and promotes a calm, focused state.

Since then, numerous other studies have shown how simple breathing exercises can create a profound shift in emotional states, helping to reduce stress in just minutes. Of course, this is also ancient knowledge that has stood the tests of time and also shows up in pretty much every culture in human history.

Shaking

A primal, animalistic reset--Shaking is your body's built-in way of discharging excess nervous system energy. Wild animals instinctively shake after stressful events to return to a state of calm, and we can too. This technique, sometimes formalized as *Neurogenic Tremoring* or *Trauma Releasing Exercises (TRE)*, is gaining popularity thanks to somatic psychology and polyvagal theory. Shaking can help regulate the autonomic nervous system, shift you out of fight/flight/freeze, and restore a sense of embodied safety. Research published in *Frontiers in Psychology* supports the use of somatic practices like TRE to reduce symptoms of trauma and anxiety. Just two minutes of shaking--literally wiggling it out--can break looping thoughts, regulate heart rate, and bring a spark of play back into the body.

Sound

Sound comes from vibration and can travel through your body in unique ways. You can use sound passively or actively to help regulate your nervous system and to help build more emotional fitness over time. Listening to music, rhythms, binaural beats, and even white noise can be soothing. Creating sound with your own voice is one of the most powerful healing tools you have access to. Chanting, humming, and other ways of creating and moving sound through the body have been used in many healing practices throughout the world for thousands of years.

Sound healing is one of my favorite tools because it can be profoundly effective in a very short time. Just two minutes of intentional sound combined with the breathing required to make it is enough to quickly recalibrate my energy most of the time.

The Shift. Own your emotions; Own your life.

Movement

In Ayurvedic medicine, it is well understood that stagnation is at the foundation of all disease. Physical movement helps with physical fitness and also helps to release emotional tension and shift energy. A study published in The Journal of Behavioral Medicine in 2002 found that regular physical activity, including light exercises like walking, significantly increases endorphin and serotonin production, leading to improved mood and reduced symptoms of anxiety and depression. Movement helps release stored emotional tension, improving both physical and emotional well-being.

Shifting Awareness

Shifting awareness involves intentionally changing our focus when emotions become overwhelming. This could mean focusing on the present moment or looking at a situation from a different angle. It could mean shifting from narrow to broad, or from near to far focus. It could mean shifting your attention more to inside your body (interoception), or more to outside our body (exteroception).

A study published in Cognitive Therapy and Research in 2004 found that cognitive shifts--moving focus away from negative thoughts--helped reduce rumination and alleviate depressive symptoms. Intentionally redirecting attention can break cycles of negative thinking and create space for positive emotions.

The Shift. Own your emotions; Own your life.

Reframing

Reframing helps us shift our perspective on difficult situations. A study in the Journal of Clinical Psychology in 2006 showed that individuals who practiced cognitive reframing techniques, which involve seeing situations from a new angle, experienced reduced emotional distress and improved emotional regulation.

By learning to reframe negative events into opportunities for growth, or change the stories we are telling ourselves about why we feel the way we do, we can enhance our emotional resilience and self-control. Remember, this does not mean deceiving ourselves or not seeing the truth. It means shifting our perspective to see a bigger picture or to see things from another point of view.

Together, these fundamental tools--pausing, questioning, breathing, moving, shifting awareness, and reframing-- equip us with practical ways to improve emotional regulation, reduce stress, and enhance self-mastery. By integrating these methods into everyday life, we train ourselves to respond to challenges with greater calm, clarity, and emotional balance.

Tapping (Emotional Freedom Technique, or EFT) is another somatic tool that combines elements of acupressure and cognitive reframing. By rhythmically tapping on specific meridian points--often starting at the side of the hand and moving through the eyebrow, under eye, chin, and collarbone--while speaking aloud a truth or reframe ("Even though I feel [emotion], I deeply and completely accept myself"), EFT helps calm the amygdala, reduce cortisol levels, and interrupt the loop of overwhelm. Multiple clinical studies, including randomized controlled trials, have shown that EFT significantly lowers symptoms of anxiety, depression, and PTSD. A 2012 study published in the *Journal of Nervous and Mental Disease* found that cortisol levels dropped by an average of 24% after a single EFT session. It's like acupressure for your emotions-- simple, fast, and no needles necessary.

A Special Note on Creativity and Art

Creative energy is one of the most underappreciated healing forces we have access to. I have found many creative practices--building, sculpting, drawing, painting, playing music, even seemingly aimless humming--all have a profound healing effect because they allow me to combine many other aspects, such as pausing, reframing, and shifting awareness or changing perspective. It also engages the senses and helps quiet the mind by narrowing focus and often can help get you back into a healthy flow cycle.

Exploring with curiosity and creating things is how we make meaning of this life. Many of us suffer from a general sense of disease that comes from not enough creative spark in our life. The great thing about that is, you can get it back anytime.

Learn to reset and recalibrate whenever you feel off, and if you are not sure where to start, creativity and art are pathways that almost always lead you back to yourself.

Not One Way

It's important to recognize that there are infinite subtle variations in how and when you can use these tools. Each of us experiences life differently, so there isn't a one-size-fits-all approach. You'll need to experiment, adapt, and practice to discover what truly works for you.

The beauty of this process is that it's yours to tailor to whatever you need. What works today may need to be adjusted tomorrow, and that's okay. Progress is fluid, not fixed.

It's also crucial to remember that personal growth isn't about doing things the 'right' way; it's about finding your way. There will be moments when the tools that work for others don't seem to fit your situation, and that's a sign that you're evolving into your own unique process.

There is no singular path to emotional regulation or self-mastery--what matters is your willingness to explore and find what resonates with you.

If you have a tool or strategy that's working well for you right now, keep using it. There's no need to change something that serves you just because there might be another option out there. However, be open to the idea that your current strategy might not always be the most effective one as you grow and evolve.

Sometimes, what we think is helping us cope is actually keeping us stuck.

This is where the distinction between *coping strategies* and *growth strategies* comes in. Coping strategies are often about managing the moment--finding ways to survive the emotional weight or stress you're feeling. These methods have value, especially in times of crisis or when you're overwhelmed. But over time, if we stay solely in coping mode, we can start to stagnate, limiting our potential for growth.

Growth strategies, on the other hand, are about pushing beyond the immediate discomfort. They're about facing challenges head-on and allowing discomfort to fuel your transformation. Remember, something can be a growth strategy at one point in your life, and a coping strategy in another. It is up to you to practice contemplating and discerning the distinctions in your own life.

Anytime you're ready, it's worth asking yourself: Am I coping, or am I growing? If you realize you've been relying on a coping strategy where a growth strategy could better serve you, that awareness itself is powerful. You don't have to make a change right away, but the moment you become conscious of it, you gain the freedom to choose differently when you're ready.

Growth isn't about abandoning what works; it's about knowing when to pivot. The tools you use today might not be the ones you need tomorrow, and that's part of the journey. Stay curious, keep experimenting, and remember that real progress is dynamic and ever-evolving.

Less Is More

One of the simplest (though not always the easiest) tools you can use is to consume less. This includes processed food and alcohol, of course, but also media, negative thoughts, and even what we currently call healthy proteins. All of these can clutter up your physical, mental, emotional, and energetic systems, leading to disease.

The Shift. Own your emotions; Own your life.

Ayurvedic medicine teaches that all disease comes from stagnation and accumulation. A universal remedy, then, is to consume less and move more. Get rid of clutter in your external and internal environment. Move, breathe, and shift your perspective. Change your diet--maybe even your hair conditioner. You might be surprised at the profound positive impact a small shift can have on your well-being.

I used to drink alcohol like it was a sport. Smoking a lot of weed and eating large portions of sugary things were also other coping strategies I used for decades. Truth be told, I may still use a couple of these old crutches now and again, though just not regularly or so excessively as I did for so many decades.

These habits served me relatively well in some ways at different points in my life, but eventually, my body started to let me know that damage was accumulating--not only from overconsumption but more acutely from allowing myself to continue 'moving forward' while increasingly out of alignment with my underlying values and beliefs.

This pattern is common in modern society and is at the heart of the emerging mental and physical health crisis. The 'fix' might be a drastic shift in behavior and environment, but it can also be a more subtle shift or a series of small changes. Usually, it's a combination of both.

Recognize that this is an individual, ongoing process. Find what works best for you right now. The first step is to stop blaming everyone else for your own misery.

Remember, your life is your responsibility. That does NOT mean being hard on yourself or beating yourself up, but it MIGHT mean demonstrating some tough love, especially at first.

The Shift. Own your emotions; Own your life.

What works best for someone else is not necessarily what will be best for you. Also, what works best for you in one phase of your life may not be what works best in another. It's all a dynamic dance and a grand experiment for you to explore within yourself.

INVITATION TO ACTION: I invite you to make a list of tools you already use to help keep yourself emotionally regulated or to help re-regulate when you get dysregulated. Which would you say are mostly coping strategies and which are growth strategies?

How often do you use them? How effective do you think they are?

Are you satisfied or pleased with the balance you have or would you like to develop or try out different coping and/or growth strategies?

Remember, there are no right or wrong answers here and as always you never have to share this with anyone, so practice being honest with yourself.

Get to Know and Love Yourself Better

A key to maximizing your effectiveness when practicing these tools is understanding your natural cycles, rhythms, and tendencies. Often, we rush through life without truly pausing to explore what makes us tick, but this exploration is essential for growth. Spend some time at the beginning of your journey really getting to know yourself--who you are beyond the noise and distractions of daily life.

Make self-awareness a regular habit, not just a passing phase. When you learn to tune in to your own needs and desires, you'll begin to treat yourself as a worthy ally rather than your own worst critic.

Start by finding ways to show yourself that you are deserving of your own love and care. Self-sabotage often comes from a place of feeling unworthy or disconnected from ourselves, so part of overcoming it is learning to build a relationship with yourself.

Figure out what truly brings you joy, what activities fill you with energy, and give yourself permission to embrace those things more fully.

This is where journaling or keeping a diary can become a powerful tool. Writing down your thoughts, emotions, and daily experiences helps you track patterns and connect with your deeper self. Over time, you'll start to see the moments when you feel your best and the habits that bring you down.

Treat yourself as someone you're genuinely curious about, as if you were meeting yourself for the first time. Take notes, keep pictures, track your feelings, and observe the nuances of your day-to-day life.

The Shift. Own your emotions; Own your life.

I'm a big fan of combining notes with pictures--it can help capture moments of happiness or growth in a more tangible way.

Chart your successes and failures, but don't judge yourself for the missteps. Instead, approach them with curiosity: what can you learn from them? As you start to see yourself more clearly, you'll have the chance to become your biggest advocate, learning to love yourself from a place of understanding and acceptance.

Convincing yourself of your own worthiness requires action. It's not enough to simply think positive thoughts; you need to actively engage in behaviors that reinforce your sense of value.

Do the things that you admire in others and feel good about doing yourself. What actions make you proud? What choices feel aligned with who you want to be? These small decisions accumulate into a greater sense of self-worth over time.

Also, don't forget the basics: assess your sleep patterns, energy levels, and daily routines. Are you getting enough rest? Do you wake up feeling energized, or are there things you could tweak to optimize your day?

Try making one or two small changes--perhaps adjusting your bedtime, incorporating a new morning ritual, or taking breaks throughout the day to recharge and try a relaxation or breathing exercise. Track how these changes affect your mood and performance.

Finally, take time to evaluate and adjust your words and actions regularly. Our self-talk plays a huge role in either reinforcing self-sabotage or fostering self-compassion. Pay attention to how you speak to yourself. Are you critical, dismissive, or harsh? If so, practice reframing those thoughts into ones that are more supportive and empowering.

Similarly, reflect on your goals and actions. Are they aligned with your values, or are you acting out of fear or habit? Try to practice compassion and patience and not blame or shame yourself or anyone else. True or not, these thoughts rev up the chemistry of dysregulation and get in your way of making clear decisions.

Learning to check in with yourself regularly will help you become your own best ally. In time you will become someone who nurtures your own growth instead of undermining it. Give yourself permission to adjust your goals and habits as you grow without shaming yourself for whatever you didn't know or get exactly right.

Balance Is Key

As you try out new tools and learn to become more of a master of your own emotions and your own life, it is important to check in with yourself regularly and make sure aspects of your life feel balanced.

Anything taken to an extreme can knock us out of balance eventually, so be on the lookout for anything that you feel very strongly about and make sure to consider other perspectives to keep yours in check.

That is not to say you can't take a strong position, it simply means that it is important to understand your own capacity and also balance your position with compassion and patience.

The Shift. Own your emotions; Own your life.

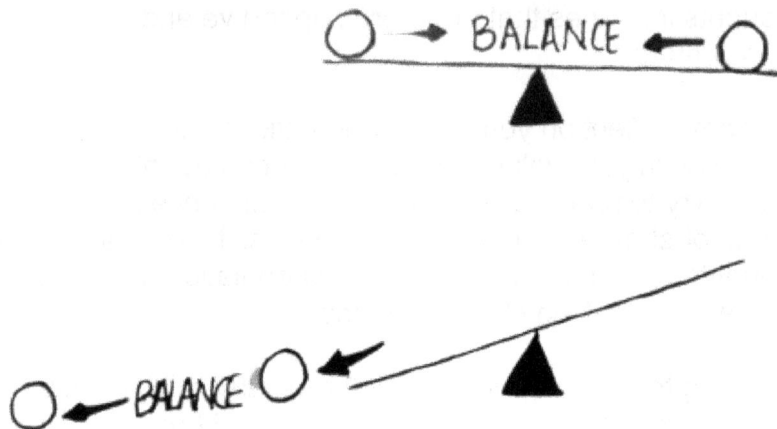

O → BALANCE ← O

O ← BALANCE O

Choosing the Tools to Keep in Your Toolkit

As you read through these tools, think about which ones
will work best in your life right now. Choose just one or two
to begin with. Give yourself time to see what works for you.
Use some method of charting or tracking your progress.
This can be as simple as a calendar with emojis or
different-colored stars, or as elaborate as a set of journals
and a 'cookie jar' of positive reminders you collect for
yourself. The point is to try things and keep the ones that
work well for you.

The most effective place to start is often with a disruption.
Then, pause or at least take your foot off the gas and
decelerate, and question. Anytime you realize or become
aware that you are repeating thoughts, ask yourself:

The Shift. Own your emotions; Own your life.

Is that really true?

How is this feeling trying to help me?

What is the polarized feeling in my subconscious that is an opportunity to be rebalanced and used as fuel rather than draining me?

Start from where you are and do the best you can with what you have. You can always upgrade as you progress. As you decide which tools to try, remember that you may need to give a new habit at least a few tries, and maybe even two or three weeks to get past that initial discomfort that comes with doing anything new. Make sure you use some method for tracking your progress.

Some of my personal tools have been useful for decades, and others have served me just for a day. If you're not seeing progress or aren't happy with the results after about three weeks, adjust, modify, or replace that tool and try something different.

When you find something that seems to unlock a new level of capacity for you, congratulate yourself. Then, take some time to really anchor it in. Evaluate what it is about that tool that works well for you so you can bring that personal insight to other tools as you build your toolkit.

If you try something you like but aren't sure it's working, keep doing it and see if you can figure out how it's helping. If any of these tools seem to make things worse, stop using that tool, at least for now, and try something else. You don't need to create a story about it, like "I hate yoga" or "I suck at meditation." Simply say to yourself, "not today" or "not for me right now," and move on.

The Basic Tools

Really the only tools any of us probably need are learning to pause--get curious and be courageous enough to ask ourselves some questions and answer ourselves more honestly. I have also found profound healing results in making changes to my diet (mainly consuming less and also focusing on healthier choices), movement patterns, slower and deeper breathing, and learning to laugh more.

Paying attention to cycles and patterns, rhythm and relaxation, play and creativity, and relationships of all sorts are also important foundational tools we all can use to increase our capacity to live more satisfying and fulfilling lives.

I currently use journaling, gratitude, mindfulness, breathwork, heart coherence, yoga, sound healing, outdoor belonging walks, snowboarding, comedy, playing music, and neurographic art as my main emotional fitness tools. I find playing music, hugs, and heartfelt conversations with friends helpful as well.

The "Pro Kit" Tools: Red, Yellow, Green Light

Basics aside, I did do a very deep dive into more than a hundred different types of healing and regulating techniques, and have them organized in alphabetical order for easy reference in a separate "Two Minute Tools" pdf you are welcome to (if you did not get a link to it with this book, please request it on my website).

For this book I have condensed this list somewhat into tools I felt were most relevant to include. I like to categorize these tools into three main groups, which I label 'red,' 'yellow,' and 'green' light tools. My hope is that you might use this section as something of a 'menu' of tools to choose from and begin by trying out one or two that sound good to you.

Red Light Tools

Red light tools are those you use in an emergency. This could be an actual emergency or a perceived one--your nervous system treats both the same. Use these tools when your fight-or-flight system is activated.

When you're overwhelmed and dysregulated, the first priority, after getting to safety, is to return to a coherent state as quickly as possible. Then, take inventory of where you are. This helps you regain coherence, anchor in the present moment, and gives you a benchmark for comparing later to see what's working and what isn't.

Over the last decade, I've started to recognize that different types of dysregulation can occur on the other side of the energetic spectrum. Euphoria, mania, or pursuing something with an extremely narrow and intense focus can also indicate that your nervous system is bypassing your higher thinking and driving you unconsciously. This is great when you're on task, in a flow state, and safe, but it can be problematic if you're not aware of being in that state. You might perceive a potential mate, partner, prize, or food source in a way that overwhelms your ability to make clear, calm, conscious choices.

For me, it's more difficult to recognize and acknowledge imbalances of positive states than of negative ones. Perhaps this has to do with my upbringing, my addictive patterns, or maybe it's a natural way of driving toward survival.

If you have an anxious, avoidant, or chaotic attachment style, or a history of neglect and/or abuse, you might be conditioned to interpret feelings of arousal or hope about love as signals of potential danger.

It's a good idea to pause before making any big decisions, especially when you feel strong emotions about it. Whether they feel extremely negative or positive, try to bring your nervous system back into a more coherent, calm state before making a choice. This is why it's often helpful to 'sleep on it' before making big decisions.

Of course, it's also important to recognize when you're actually in an emergency or under real threat. In these times, you're likely to respond more effectively if you practice using the same tools you'd use when misinterpreting 'false' threats as real ones.

Emergencies and feelings of extreme urgency can flip most of us almost instantly into a sympathetic state, bypassing our logical minds and connecting our actions and words directly to our limbic system. This is a healthy and natural survival mechanism. It's very difficult, if not impossible, to think at all--let alone 'think straight'--when we're in this 'fight or flight' state.

This state arises when your system determines that you need to take fast, extraordinary action. It could be that you really are in danger or in a position to help someone else in immediate danger. It could be that something you desire is within your immediate grasp, and a moment of hesitation could cost you what you want. Assessing the situation is something you can train yourself to get better at with practice.

After you're out of immediate danger, or if you determine that your system is being activated when you're not actually in danger--either due to our modern hyper-stimulating environment, your personal surroundings, or a hypervigilant, traumatized, or overactivated system--the next priority is to regain calm coherence. THEN choose and implement your responses with more of your full faculties at hand.

Learn to recognize when you're dysregulated and reset your system. This is a technique used by the military and other institutions that understand human performance. It can be highly effective.

If you're in immediate danger, keeping your nervous system as calm as possible is still usually going to give you the best chance of survival.

Modern life tends to trigger a sense of dread or existential threat, even when we're not in actual immediate danger. Just two minutes of listening to advertising or 'news' on television or radio is enough to activate a partially threatened state in most of us.

The Shift. Own your emotions; Own your life.

Many people are currently living in a nearly perpetual state of existential threat. Our systems become chaotic and start to break down when they're incoherent for too long. Finding ways to reset your nervous system and regain coherence is increasingly challenging and necessary. Regularly disengage or unplug from our modern, overstimulating environment. This is a healthy strategy. Make it a regular practice, and you'll feel better.

The Red light tools that I currently keep in my toolkit are:

Physiological Sigh: is a science-backed breath technique that's as quick as it is effective. It involves two short inhales through the nose (one deep, one topping it off) followed by a slow, extended exhale through the mouth. This method was studied by Dr. Andrew Huberman and colleagues at Stanford, who found it to be the most efficient breathing pattern for rapidly reducing stress and restoring calm. It works by offloading carbon dioxide and increasing lung inflation, which activates pulmonary stretch receptors that cue the parasympathetic nervous system (the "rest and digest" mode). Even one or two cycles can help reset the body after a stress spike—like a literal sigh of relief, but supercharged.

Pause: When you feel overwhelmed, simply stop. Take a moment to bring awareness to your state.

Questions: Ask yourself, "Is this really true?" or "How can I reframe this situation?"

Breath: Use deep, calming breaths to bring your nervous system back to a more regulated state.

The Shift. Own your emotions; Own your life.

Bounce: Physical movement, like gentle bouncing, can help shift your energy.

Hum: Vibrating the vagus nerve can help reset the nervous system and bring you back to a calmer state.

Sway: Swaying from side to side can have a calming effect on the body.

Sigh: A deep, intentional sigh can release tension.

Sing: Singing can help to re-regulate your emotional state.

Movement in Space: Moving around your environment, even just a little, can change your state.

Shake it off: Literally shaking your body can help reset your nervous system.

Forward Locomotion: Moving forward, even if just mentally envisioning it, can help shift your perspective.

Touching Hands: Self-soothing through physical touch, like rubbing your hands together or placing a hand on your heart, can be grounding.

Checking Basic Needs: Ensure you're not hungry, thirsty, or in need of sleep.

The Flip: Mentally flipping your perspective on a situation can provide new insights. Check in with your thoughts and see if your thinking is creating a trauma response in your body. If it is, congratulate yourself for catching this and see if you can use the momentum of this to reconnect to your values, your goals, and your mission. Use it as a prompt to remember what is really important to you and make sure your thoughts and actions are aligning with that.

The Shift. Own your emotions; Own your life.

Cold Water: A splash of cold water on your face, a cool shower, or even drinking a glass of cold water can be a great way to quickly reset your nervous system.

Recognize Dysregulation and Then Pause-Breathe-Question

One of the most critical skills you can develop is learning to recognize when your body is dysregulated or in the process of becoming dysregulated. Dysregulation can manifest as a sense of internal incoherence--like you're no longer in sync with yourself--or as a subtler feeling of turbulence under the surface. When you're dysregulated, your body's systems--heart rate, breath, muscle tension--begin to shift out of their natural rhythm, often leading to a flood of emotions that can cloud your ability to think clearly and make rational decisions.

Pay attention to physical cues: Is your heart rate accelerating? Has your breathing become shallow or rapid? Do you feel a tightness in your chest or stomach, a lump in your throat, cold hands, tingling, or heat rising in your body? These are common signals that your system is dysregulated or becoming dysregulated, and they are your invitation to pause, breathe, and take notice. It's important to catch these moments early, as allowing dysregulation to persist often leads to reactive behavior--such as snapping at someone, making impulsive decisions, or shutting down emotionally--before you even realize what's happening.

The first step to resetting is almost always to shift your attention inward and bring awareness to your breath. If you are already focused on your internal function and sensing extreme anxiety or panic, it can be helpful to shift your attention outward and notice objects of a certain color or count the round objects you can see, for example.

226

The Shift. Own your emotions; Own your life.

In moments of acute dysregulation, it can help to exhale deeply before trying to take a full, calming breath. This signals to your body that it's safe to begin the process of calming down. Once your breathing begins to slow and deepen, you'll find it easier to ask yourself helpful questions like: "What am I really feeling right now?" or "Is this reaction serving me?"

When dysregulation interferes with your ability to navigate situations rationally, it's because the brain's fight-or-flight response hijacks your thinking processes. When the nervous system senses a perceived threat--whether it's a difficult conversation, an emotional trigger, or physical discomfort--it prepares for survival. This triggers a chemical cascade which can leave you feeling emotionally overwhelmed or mentally scattered. Your logical brain, responsible for clear reasoning and decision-making, temporarily takes a backseat.

This is why it's so important to re-regulate before making choices or reacting. Trying to act rationally when you're dysregulated is like trying to row a tiny boat against the current of a huge ocean in a storm--you need to wait for the storm to pass, get your bearings, assess your situation, and then get back on course as quickly as possible.

In my own experience, the first thing I often notice when I'm dysregulated is difficulty breathing or a tightness in my throat or chest. My breath becomes shallow, and sometimes I start to tear up or feel flushed and agitated. Sometimes my heart races or I get a wave of anxiety. Sometimes my hands tingle or feel cold.

These are clear signals that my body is out of balance, and they remind me to shift my focus. I've learned that when I pause and concentrate on bringing my breath back to a steady rhythm, the rest of my body--and my mind--can follow suit. From this more coherent state, I can think more clearly, make decisions that align with my true intentions, and respond to the world from a place of calm rather than reactivity.

Learning to recognize dysregulation and respond to it with tools like pause-breathe-question is essential. It allows you to stay connected to your rational mind, even in the face of emotional turbulence. With practice, you'll begin to see these moments not as setbacks but as opportunities to reset and approach life with more clarity and intentionality.

Yellow Light Tools

When I've made big decisions, I find it helpful to pretend I've made a choice, sleep on it, and check in with my nervous system first thing in the morning. Waking up to a new choice can feel exciting, or it can fill you with dread. It's helpful to give it a trial run if you can before 'signing on the dotted line' or committing yourself to something that might not align with your core values, even if you can't quite put your finger on why at the time.

This isn't to say you'll never have to move forward in doubt. Many times, we simply can't know how things will work out. When you look back on your life, most of the decisions you make probably won't matter much. Keep in mind that goals are vehicles to help you become more of the person you want to be. The destination itself can be arbitrary.

Of course, the reason our systems sometimes respond with rapid shifts in neurochemistry is that sometimes we do need to take fast action. Wasting precious time on logic can cost us the prize or even our lives. There are times when pausing and questioning isn't an appropriate response.

Fortunately, this is our default setting, so unless you've trained for deep diving or other extreme abilities to override your nervous system, you're likely to respond to 'predators' and 'prey' automatically. Evaluating the difference takes practice, and you'll get better at it the more you do it.

In real-time, you're not likely to have time to think through "Is this a red, yellow, or green light situation?" when it's a red-light situation. Learn to recognize the signs of dysregulation in your body. Take immediate action to re-regulate your system to the best of your ability as soon as you do.

Your body has this system built in to help keep you alive in dangerous situations and to help you 'get the prize' when it's in reach. Mating and finding food are just as important as avoiding predators and taking shelter from storms when it comes to basic survival.

With practice, you can develop your skill of recognizing and more accurately assessing your own emotional state and start to notice when others are dysregulated. When others are dysregulated, it's not a good time to try to work things out. It's usually not a good time to come to an agreement about something, other than perhaps agreeing to breathe or move together to come back into coherence. After regulation is reestablished, you'll find your efforts lead to much greater progress.

Try not to spend time going around in trauma loops or revving up the dysregulation with negative thoughts. Make an agreement with yourself that you'll do your best to shift the next time you notice any signs or sensations indicating dysregulation. Don't beat yourself up when you realize

The Shift. Own your emotions; Own your life.

you're not doing as well as you'd like. Instead, congratulate yourself for recognizing it, and adjust accordingly.

Remember, the point is not to complicate things or create friction, except to the degree that we need to pattern interrupt sometimes. The point is to develop a system of organizing your tools so that you know what to do, and which tool to use, in any given situation--automatically, without thinking about it.

It merits another reminder here that resistance is like glue to the things we resist. Rather than pushing against the thing or idea you don't want, put your attention on what you DO want. Let your resistance fade.

In time, you may even come to genuinely appreciate when you recognize resistance in your body or energy. This is a clue that there's growing dissonance or tension between your ant and the elephant, and/or the 'room' you're in.

Check in with yourself and ask your body and your spirit or soul or energetic self what it needs. Remember to speak to yourself gently, like someone you want to feel and act lovingly towards.

The Yellow Light Tools I keep in my toolkit are all the Red Light Tools, plus

Journaling—I write down my dreams and plans every morning, as well as process anything that is bothering me and track several other things. I also keep a more brief gratitude and accomplishment journal that I write in nearly every night as I am getting ready for bed. I write down things only that make me feel good in that journal. Numerous studies and countless personal accounts evidence that journaling may be one of the most widely used and effective tools to develop more self-awareness and emotional fitness over time.

Painting relaxes me and helps me express my feelings in ways that words can't. I love the language of colors and lines, of forms and juxtapositions. There is a growing body of research in the field of art therapy to help explain what humans have long known intuitively, which is that color, texture, symbols, lines, juxtaposition, timing and contrast are all wonderful tools for self-expression and processing our often complex emotions and feelings.

Doodling or Cartooning—sometimes making a cartoon or just doodling about my feelings helps me see them in a different light and process them in a healthy way. Again, this is an excellent and credible way to explore and express your emotions and develop your emotional fitness.

Deep Breathing—deep, slow breathing calms the body, and when I practice it regularly it helps me stay more regulated even when I am not doing it at the time. Regular deep breathing exercises are one of the best things you can do for my body, mind, and spirit. It's also free and easy and available any time.

Stretching is another wonderful practice that can improve your mental, physical, and emotional health. Stretching is a foundational part of my personal emotional and physical fitness routine.

Sound Healing/Humming/Singing—Sound healing has been a favorite tool in my tool box since I was young—humming and singing and talking to myself. Now we understand more about the vagus nerve and how vibrating our vocal chords helps to build vagal tone, which is directly correlated to our degree of emotional fitness. This is an exciting field where new research is again confirming what humans have long known. The power of sound is an exciting, largely untapped resource for healing and expression.

Belonging Walks is what I call getting outside and remembering that I belong exactly where I am, that I am part of this earth, and also sometimes connect with my neighbors and many of the animals in my neighborhood. Again, there is good research to show that being outdoors, or even thinking about nature can improve our internal chemistry. Our sense of belonging is also crucial to our overall sense of wellbeing. I find walking outside and remembering I am a part of this earth, along with the birds and the trees and the bees, helps me to feel connected to life in a way that helps me navigate the dramas of human society more calmly and coherently.

Talking to friends and/or sometimes 'strangers'- It's good to have a friend to talk to. My brain sometimes tries to tell me I don't have any real friends, but then I realize this is not true. I actually have many great people in my life, and we are all doing our best to the best humans we can be. Getting an outside perspective is often helpful if I am having trouble processing something.

Comedy—Laughter is truly great medicine, so I regularly find a great stand-up comedy act, occasionally try to make my own, and recently am beginning to explore Laughter Yoga. Really, if you could only choose one tool from this entire book, laughter would probably be the best choice.

Exaggeration—making fun of my own drama and really allowing myself to fully embrace a pity party for a short time often helps snap me out of it. Sometimes I sing a silly song: *"POOOOOR Me. Nobody loves me—Might as well go eat some worms…shit I ain't got no worms…Ooooh Weellll."*

The Shift. Own your emotions; Own your life.

Vagal Toning—I use humming and specific vocal exercises to help increase the tone of my vagus nerve, which has been shown to have a significant effect on how well we handle stress and how well we return to a regulated state when we do become dysregulated.

Green Light Tools

Many of us have been trained to override our natural guidance systems to such an extent that we don't notice the signs and signals until dysregulation becomes intense. We may have been living in a chronically dysregulated state for so long that we think this is normal.

Often, we only pay attention to our emotional overwhelm when it reaches a full-blown meltdown, rendering us unable to function. It can be tricky to recognize the difference between building resilience and suppression/repression, especially at the beginning of this journey towards more emotional mastery.

Many of us are told we have excess emotions because we are damaged or defective. We may be convinced that we should numb ourselves or choose from a menu of questionable drugs. This can create a narrative of ongoing or permanent disability.

It can also create a cascade of immune responses, mood swings, stagnation and accumulations in the body. Cultivating emotional resilience requires learning to process all our different emotions in healthier ways. It does not mean feeling less, or even less intensely. It does take practice, however, just like developing physical strength takes regular training.

The Shift. Own your emotions; Own your life.

Neurodivergence, with labels such as Autism, Dyslexia, and ADHD; PTSD and generational trauma; and growing up in a family or culture that shuns emotions are all factors that can make it extra challenging to develop the skills we need to navigate emotions in healthy ways. Some of us may feel our emotions more intensely than others.

Hormonal fluctuations and life changes can make use extra sensitive and decrease our bandwidth or capacity to handle challenges.

It can be helpful to have a reason, a diagnosis, a story that helps us put the question of "what is happening" more to ease. Whatever the reason, though, see if you can suspend that belief instead of using it as an excuse, and practice regulation instead of fueling your self-limiting beliefs.

Regulation is a skill you can learn and improve, regardless of what else is going on in and around you. Yes, there are internal and external factors at play. Most of them are out of your control. Focus on the factors you can control.

Quit telling yourself the same negative story and try out new strategies until you find something that works. You might be more sensitive, you might need extra outside help, but that probably means you have extra potential to rise and shine too. Remember, this is your life, and your life is no one else's responsibility.

If this resonates with you, I encourage you to go slow, be patient with yourself. Recognize that the people you keep in your life are highly likely to be in a similar energetic state as you, and together you are likely repeating the same patterns and trauma loops. This doesn't mean they are trying to hurt you or mean you harm—far from it—but it does mean they might not be helping you, and you might not be helping them.

You may need to spend a period of time in some degree of isolation, cocooning yourself so you can develop new regulation skills.

As you practice taking responsibility for your own emotional state, you'll become more able to interact with specific people or scenarios without being triggered into an emotional reaction. Those areas that cause regular meltdowns or high-energy reactions are likely the places where you're most out of alignment with your values. Pay attention to any area where you notice this is the case.

The point of all this is to say, Green Light Tools are in many ways the most difficult to implement sometimes.

It can take a long time to change your relationship to food or to family or co-workers, or to yourself. It takes time to change your health if you have spent a long time indulging less than healthy habits and built momentum in the opposite direction. It can be difficult, and it can take time; but also, it can be done.

In addition to the Red and Yellow Light Tools, the Green Light Tools I currently keep in my toolkit are:

- Regular practice of Yoga and Meditation
- Joining a gym and/or working out regularly
- Improving my relationships with my mother, my son, people I play music with, myself, my neighbors, pretty much everyone I see or meet, and with

humanity at large, with my own spirit, and with this earth.
- Getting out of debt and putting money into savings
- Getting out of town regularly for kayaking, snowboarding, or rock hunting, hiking…something!
- Hot and cold showers daily
- A regimen of herbs and vitamins
- Eating plenty of healthy protein, fats, and vegetables and not too much processed food, including sugar and simple carbohydrates
- Belonging to a community or group-We are communal creatures, like it or not. Our brains and bodies do best when we are around other people regularly. I try to get around other humans several times a week. At times in my life this has been much more, and at other times less. I play music with a couple of different groups, have supper with my son, lunch with my mother, and trips to the mountains and lakes whenever I can.
- Vagus nerve toning through sound healing.

It can be painful and taxing to do this work--the work of self improvement and cultivating more fitness and freedom in my life. I have great compassion for those who choose not to, as it is currently easier in many ways to go along with the dysfunctions of society. The only things harder than doing the work of self-mastery, in my eyes, is not doing it, and living a life of mediocrity knowing I didn't even try.

Taking on too much is another way we can keep ourselves looping in a lower energetic state. **It's not our job to fix the world or save anyone else. It is our job to take the best care of ourselves that we can and help others when we are able.** We can be more helpful to others when we take care of ourselves first.

The Shift. Own your emotions; Own your life.

It's true that too much of this way of thinking can lead us to be stuck in the 'savior complex' or the martyr side of the low-flying disk I mentioned earlier. If you realize you're using caring for others as an excuse not to take good care of yourself, simply pause, exhale, and shift yourself into a higher energetic state.

You don't have to carry the weight of the world on your shoulders to take responsibility for your own life. There is a lot of room for variability in this. Do what you can. Heal what you can. Improve what you can. Let the rest go.

I want to add, this does not mean that the mundane and everyday things do not create meaning in our lives. Quite the contrary. The everyday, regular, mundane aspects make up the majority of our lives. Hopefully there will be some spectacular moments of Ole' and Bravo and Big Magic too.

The Shift to take personal responsibility and develop more emotional fitness will help you enjoy all of those moments-- the mundane and the exceptional. You can uplevel every aspect of your life by choosing to be the master of your own destiny and your own life--day to day, moment to moment, story to story.

Human history has ample evidence that individuals do make a significant difference. In any case, I seem to be drawn with very large shoulders and wired with an exceptional drive to DO something. I have a strong drive to help and actively participate in this life. In my younger years, I used this as an excuse to ignore healthy boundaries and wound up damaging myself and my relationships.

The Shift. Own your emotions; Own your life.

Reviewing the Tools & Choosing the Best Ones for You

Pause & Breathe

The first tool I nearly always use is the Pause, usually followed immediately by bringing my attention to my breath. The "physiological sigh," as it's called, involves taking a deep breath in, followed by a second, smaller inhale to fully inflate the lungs, holding briefly, and then exhaling through the mouth. Sometimes, it takes a few rounds of slow, deep box breathing to gain enough control before adding the sigh at the top of the inhale, hold, and exhale.

Bringing attention to my breath also creates that essential pause, allowing me to check in with what the narrator in my head is saying. Often, I find that a fearful or victim-state default program is running.

Question Your Own "Authority"

Anytime you notice a repetitive or negative thought, see if you can interrupt the pattern. Don't automatically believe what you think. Ask yourself one or all of the following questions:

"What is really true?"

"Is that really true?"

"Is that the whole and only truth?"

"How is it serving me to think about this right now?"

238

The Shift. Own your emotions; Own your life.

"Can I do anything about that from here and now?"

"What can I think about to help bring myself back to a more regulated state?"

Sometimes, your internal narrator will answer "Yes" to the "Is it really true?" question and start justifying the thought even more. At this point, ask again, this time with a bit more determination, something such as, "Are you sure that's the complete truth, the only truth, and nothing but the truth?"

Be genuinely curious if you can. This approach is particularly useful for those dysfunctional patterns that recur in your life. By getting curious and inquiring within, you can untangle underlying unconscious or outdated beliefs that are no longer serving you. These are often the things that create chronic dysregulation in our lives.

If you can hold yourself in the potential space created by the pause, you'll begin to unravel your brain's hold on the thought. You may find you're able to put even more space around it with questions like, "Why do I think I think that?", "How would I feel if I didn't think that?", or "How is it serving me to believe that?"

A crucial component of this exercise is understanding that re-regulation is priority one. If my body is unsafe, or if the dysregulation is due to some physical factor, I need to address that right away. If it is due to my own thinking, then I can shift my thinking with deliberate thoughts. If I can't seem to do that for myself, I use default programming that I know can help re-regulate me, such as music, comedy, or one of my favorite podcasts.

Remember, this is purely for you. You don't need to share it with anyone else, and it's not helpful to be dishonest or hide things from yourself in this process. Most people find that writing, drawing, or even interpretive dancing without overthinking is helpful in getting to the subconscious truths of what's really going on. Try not to overanalyze. Remember, there isn't just one way to do this. Find what works for you and simply let go of anything that doesn't.

Your Basic Needs Are Your Responsibility

To put this another way, your ability to respond is dependent on you taking care of your own basic needs. If you have trouble with this then put support systems in place to make sure you get the basic bases covered. When you notice dysregulation in your body one of your responses ought to be to check in with your basic biological needs. What do you need? What is your body trying to tell you?

Remember that emotions are merely data, and feelings are the story you're making up about that data, which is likely to be inaccurate or incomplete. Rather than dive into the story, try to just notice the physical sensations in your body and think about what they could be communicating. Get curious before you start to tell yourself stories about what your emotions mean.

A good place to start is almost always to check in on your body's basic needs for food, water, and safety. If you have spent a lot of time disassociating from your body, you might be surprised to learn that a good deal of the dysregulation you are experiencing can be fixed by routinely taking care of your basic needs. Check in with your basic needs early and often throughout this process.

Is your glucose low?

How about your electrolytes? Do you need a pinch of mineral-rich salt in your water?

Are you thirsty, or do you need to pee?

Have you been drinking enough clean water?

How is your sleep lately?

241

The Shift. Own your emotions; Own your life.

Where are you in your hormonal cycle?

How much have you been exercising lately?

When was the last time you danced?

When was the last time you sang, hummed, or used your voice to make a beat?

How well are you managing your stress levels lately?

Do you need some extra recovery time?

Is your body dealing with extra stimulation that you haven't been mindful of and so aren't managing well?

By identifying reasons you may be feeling dysregulated, you can create a reinforcing safety loop, letting your body know that caring for your basic needs is something you're always going to do to the best of your ability.

Be sure to take positive action once you've identified something you think might be part of 'the problem.' Sometimes I spend a lot of time contemplating the problem, come to a potential solution, and then still don't take any action. This can propagate that feeling of self-sabotage and lead to more negative spiraling. If you find yourself doing this, pause, get up, and take positive action.

Drink some water.

Go outside and exhale.

Give yourself two minutes to breathe and stretch.

The Shift. Own your emotions; Own your life.

Take your vitamins or herbs.

Hug a friend or give yourself a hug.

Put on a good song and sing along.

Dance! Laugh!

Do the thing that you've concluded is likely to help. It probably will, and you'll gain positive momentum with more practice. Remember, just start where you are and do the best you can.

Once you make this inventory, take the necessary steps to remedy the immediate causes if possible. If it's not possible to give your body what it needs right away, make a note and assure yourself that you will as soon as you can. Remind yourself that this situation will change eventually and resolve to get through it as best as you can.

If it seems unbearable or impossible, or you find yourself repeating the same self-defeating story, you might need to do some work. Journal or create some art with genuine curiosity. See if you can discover something new about yourself.

If you really can't bring yourself to do the work and feel better because you're feeling overwhelmed, choose a healthy distraction like comedy or gazing at clouds in the sky. Compartmentalize whatever it is for the time being if you can and focus on something that you can control.

Patterns, Rhythm, Movement, and Disruption

One of the most effective ways to calm your nervous system and bring your body back into coherence is through patterns, rhythm, and subtle disruption. Establishing a pattern--whether through counting, tapping, drumming, or even just paying attention to your breath--can quickly balance the two halves of your brain and regulate your body's biochemistry.

Something as simple as counting your steps or focusing on your breathing can be a first step toward calming down an overstimulated nervous system. You could try noticing your heartbeat or listening to an external sound that follows a rhythm. The key is to find what works best for you and use it to bring yourself into a more balanced, coherent state.

When energy is built up in your body, shaking, tapping, patting, rubbing, or even more subtle forms of movement can help dissipate that energy and restore calm. Whether it's a gentle sway, rocking back and forth, or something more vigorous like shaking your arms or legs, these movements can help your nervous system find its way back to equilibrium.

The goal is to experiment with different techniques, listen to your body, and find what works in the moment. We are incredibly adaptable creatures, capable of tuning into our physical sensations and using movement as a powerful tool to self-regulate.

Movement isn't just about large, dramatic gestures. Sometimes the most subtle and gentle movements can have the most profound impact. Realigning your posture, for example, can shift your energetic state. When you feel low or stressed, your body naturally collapses inward— shoulders hunch, the spine curls, the head drops.

The Shift. Own your emotions; Own your life.

By consciously lifting your chin, straightening your spine, and aligning your body, you send a signal to your nervous system that you're resuming a regulated, balanced state. It's a simple yet powerful way to bring yourself back online.

The Shift. Own your emotions; Own your life.

Tapping, Touch, Temperature

Tapping uses rhythm and touch to help regulate the nervous system. There are different methods such as the Emotional Freedom Technique (EFT) and in some qi gong and martial arts warm up practices. Many healing techniques use some form of rhythmic tapping or counting.

Touch is another crucial tool for emotional regulation, though one that is often neglected in modern society. Many of us were not only deprived of healthy, nurturing touch as children but may have also experienced harmful or confusing touch. This can leave us with nervous systems that find touch challenging, if not triggering. It's essential to reframe touch as a source of safety and comfort, especially when it comes to self-soothing.

A self-hug, gentle tapping, or even pressing your palms together can be incredibly soothing. Wrapping yourself in a soft blanket or grounding yourself by focusing on where your body is supported by the earth can also help. The key is to experiment with different forms of touch to see what resonates with you.

You might find that pressing your body into a corner or using firm touch, like placing your hands on your chest, helps bring you back to center. Touch can also be a great way to redirect your body's attention through changes in temperature--try using a hot or cold pack, or even tapping or slapping lightly to reset your nervous system.

Temperature is another great tool that most of us can use any time to help reset and also build more resilience in the nervous system. Splashing cold water on your face, washing your hands in cold or hot water, a hot or cold shower, a heat or ice pack, cold plunges, saunas, and other methods are all ways that humans have figured out to

246

help us cultivate more self-mastery, specifically in the way of physical, psychological, emotional, and neurological fitness.

Learning to use touch as a self-regulation tool empowers you to soothe your body without relying on others. By bringing awareness to where you feel sensations in your body and naming those sensations, you help your nervous system organize itself, moving from chaos to coherence.

Sound Healing and Vibration

Sound is another tool that can have a profound impact on our emotional and physical state. Whether it's the steady rhythm of a drum, the ringing of a bell, or the hum of your own voice, sound vibrations easily permeate the body and influence our nervous system. Instruments like singing bowls, gongs, or even blowing into a horn or conch shell can have a deeply calming effect. You might even experiment with Baoding balls or simply listening to your favorite music. I use sound healing as a red, yellow, and green light tool.

It's important to recognize the role that sound plays in your regulation process. Is the music or sound you're engaging with helping you re-regulate and bring coherence, or is it simply distracting you from your dysregulation? Both can serve a purpose, but if you find yourself relying more on distraction than true healing, it might be time to re-evaluate your strategies and upgrade your toolkit.

Vibrating the vagus nerve has been shown to help tonify the entire nervous system and also create measurable changes in many of the hormones and neurochemicals that are known to effect our emotional states the most, such as

The Shift. Own your emotions; Own your life.

dopamine, oxytocin, serotonin, epinephrine, cortisol, and nitric oxide. There is a growing body of exciting research in this field, and a wide array of exercises and tools you can use starting right now.

INVITATION TO ACTION: I invite you to explore making some sound and vibrating your vagus nerve, which runs through the center of your body and connects your brain, your voice box, your digestive system, your heart, and more. A simple sound you can start with is *"AAAAOOOOMMMM." [This represents the beginning, middle, and end and makes a soothing meditative chant]*.

You can choose any sound or word, preferably something with a consonant and a vowel. There are specific sounds [Eem, Aam, Aim, Aom, Om, Oom, Um; Sa, Ta, Na, Ma] used in chakra healing and in other practices but it is not necessary to get specific in the beginning.

If you like, place your hands gently on your neck or along your jaw line and notice the vibrations as you generate sound in your own body. Repeat this five or ten times, gaining volume if you can without forcing or straining your voice. Try to relax your throat and breathe deeper and slower. After a minute or two, check in with your body and notice how you feel. Do you feel any different from before the exercise?

The Power of Disruption

While soothing techniques like rhythm, touch, and sound are important for restoring calm, sometimes what's needed is a more abrupt interruption to your system. A sudden jolt, like a quick slap to the body, a cold splash of water, or even an electromagnetic shock, can quickly shift you out of a dysregulated state. These disruptions work by shocking the nervous system into recalibration, forcing it to reorganize and come back to balance.

It's important, though, to have a desired outcome in mind when using these techniques. Whether it's returning to a state of calm, refocusing on a task, or simply feeling more centered, having a clear, prioritized outcome will help your body and mind recalibrate more effectively. Once you've reset, you can then practice shifting into a more productive emotional state and taking coherent, aligned actions.

The goal is to build a custom toolkit for emotional regulation that works for you. The tools you choose--whether they involve movement, sound, touch, or disruption--should help you cultivate coherence and balance in your life. The better you become at managing your internal state, the quicker you'll be able to take meaningful, aligned actions that move you toward the life you desire.

Using Your Body and All Its Senses

Think about all your senses and all the ways your body takes in data--from sight, touch, smell, and sound, to proprioception and interoception, balance, temperature, and gravity. Any shift you can create in the data being processed can potentially shift you into a more regulated state.

The Shift. Own your emotions; Own your life.

Remember that, usually, unless there is actual immediate danger you need to respond to, you'll do best to find a soothing, non-destructive, perhaps even healthy shift, rather than merely disrupting. Again, though, sometimes any disruption can create or begin to create a positive shift and open a space to shift into a more coherent state.

When I'm playing my guitar and I break a string or it goes drastically out of tune during a song, I adjust immediately by playing that string less and tuning it in the song if I can. At the soonest opportunity, I stop the regular flow of the show to fix the issue because it's too far out of tune or broken to continue. If need be, I remove the string and continue to play until the next break, then put on a new string or switch guitars, or do whatever is necessary. If the guitar is only slightly out of tune, I'll wait until between songs or even wait for a break a few more songs in to tune it up. Then there's regular tuning and practice.

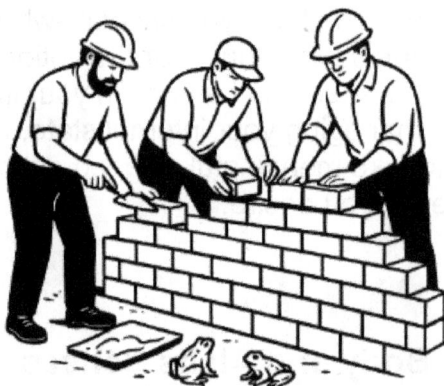

The Parable of the Three Builders

In a bustling town, not very long ago, three builders worked on a grand construction site, each laying bricks under the heat of the sun. A curious traveler passed by and asked each builder the same simple question: "What are you doing?"

The first builder, weary and covered in dust, sighed and said, "I'm just laying bricks. One at a time, day after day. It's hard work, and it never seems to end." He worked slowly, resentfully placing each brick down with little care, focusing only on getting through the long hours of labor.

The traveler moved on to the second builder, who had a more thoughtful air about him. "I'm building a wall," he said with a touch of pride. His work was steady and methodical, and while his task was still challenging, he understood that it had a greater purpose than simply laying bricks. He took satisfaction in seeing the wall rise, one brick at a time.

Finally, the traveler approached the third builder. This man was humming to himself, his eyes bright with enthusiasm as he worked. "What are you doing?" the traveler asked.

The third builder smiled broadly and said, "I'm building a cathedral! Every brick I lay, no matter how small, is part of something far bigger and more magnificent than myself. This cathedral will stand for generations to come, and I'm proud to be a part of its creation."

Though all three builders were engaged in the same physical task, their perspectives were worlds apart. The first saw his work as mundane and draining, the second found purpose in the immediate task at hand, and the third

251

had a vision far beyond the daily grind--one that inspired him to approach even the smallest tasks with energy and purpose.

In the same way, if we can shift our perspective from focusing solely on the immediate task to embracing a bigger vision, we begin to see how every small step matters. Each brick, no matter how insignificant it might seem in the moment, is part of the larger structure we are building in our lives. By aligning our habits with our larger goals, we not only make progress but create quantum leaps--moments of exponential growth that come from consistent, focused effort over time.

It's easy to think that quantum leaps require drastic, dramatic changes, but the truth is, they often come from the consistent accumulation of small, well-placed actions. The difference lies in how we perceive and approach those actions. Are we just laying bricks, or are we building cathedrals? The shift is internal and often seem subtle from the outside, but the results are significant--instantly and over time.

By shifting our mindset to see the cathedral, we turn every small habit into a building block for something greater. The atomic habits--small, deliberate steps--become part of the foundation that supports a quantum leap in progress. With this broader perspective, even the most routine actions gain meaning and significance. We begin to see how each task, each habit, is part of a much larger journey toward our goals and dreams.

TO GET ALL YOUR DUCKS, IN A ROW, YOU'VE GOT TO JUST GO!

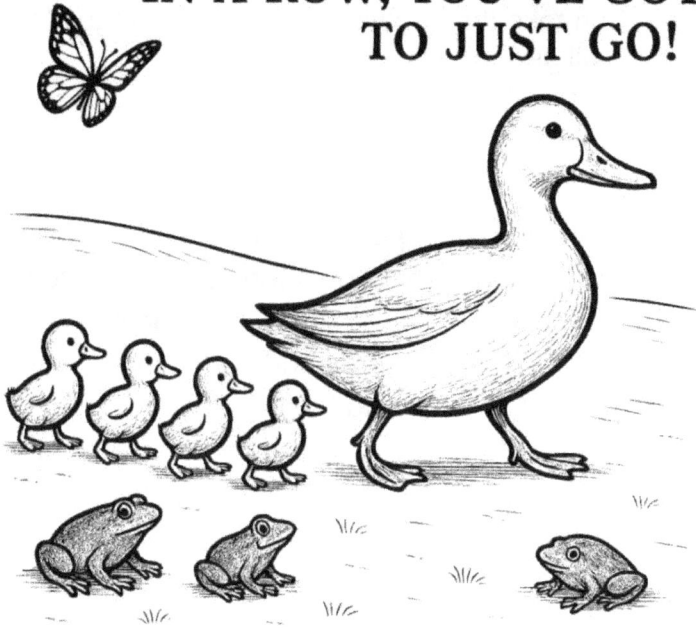

You can't actually get ducks in a row by waiting. You must waddle forward, and then you'll find all your ducklings will naturally fall in line.

Any tool you find that works for you is wise to keep in your toolkit. Remember, there is not 'one way' to heal, and there is not one way to make a fantastic life. Try new things until you find something that works, then practice that to see if it improves.

If nothing seems to work, that is usually a sign that your basic needs and sense of safety are so threatened that your body needs to stay in the parasympathetic system in order to best survive. If you recognize that you are not in real danger and your system has established a dysfunctional pattern, take heart, brave one, for this is a good sign that you are making progress on your healing journey. Then take the necessary steps to re-regulate yourself. It will get easier with practice.

INVITATION TO ACTION: Write down three of the tools that sparked enough interest in you to consider trying. Think about when or how you might practice using each tool and jot down any pros and cons that come to mind when you consider using the tool in your life. Choose at least one of the tools and make an action plan to give it a try.

Summary of Chapter Five

You can shift your perspective. You can change your breathing. You can almost always shift your posture or your focus, thereby shifting your energetic state. This can make a huge difference. Remember that everything is temporary, and ride it out the best you can. Simply adding more order to your situation in any way you can--with a rhythm or a soothing pattern--can help bring your parasympathetic nervous system back 'online.'

When you realize you are feeling dysregulated, try not to spend your energy blaming anyone else or shaming yourself. Pause, question, breathe, and check in with your basic needs. Then use one or two of the tools you have found that work best for you.

Count backwards from 100. Try some music. Take a walk. Do some yoga. Call a friend or strike up a conversation with someone at a bus stop. Tune in to nature and listen to the birds and bugs that are busily taking care of themselves. Get inspired and create something.

Once you are feeling more regulated, evaluate the situation and see if there are things that need more adjustment. Maybe you need a new hobby. Maybe you need to clean the kitchen. Maybe you need a new job or a vacation. Try not to make any big decisions from a dysregulated state.

Remember that sometimes survival is the highest form of self-care. Check in with your behaviors and the stories you are telling yourself to be sure you are not actually harming yourself and calling it self-care. If you are feeling threatened and believe you need to defend yourself with the vim and vigor appropriate for a life-threatening situation--when it's actually just a 'leaf in the sky' or some other misinterpreted data--you may cause yourself or others harm by existing in 'survival mode' when you could be healing or developing new skills.

More Real People Who Inspire Me:

Peter Sage's Story: Turning Adversity into Opportunity

Peter Sage's story is one of navigating setbacks and using challenges as opportunities to refine one's personal toolkit. In 2017, after a series of legal battles, Peter was sentenced to six months in Pentonville Prison for contempt of court. For many people, prison could have been a devastating blow, but Peter chose to approach it with a mindset of personal growth and service. He refused to let the external situation dictate his internal experience.

Instead of viewing his imprisonment as a punishment, Peter treated it as a learning experience and an opportunity to apply his personal development tools. He began to mentor other inmates, offering them guidance on mindset, emotional regulation, and personal empowerment. His unique approach led to profound changes, not only in himself but in the lives of many others he encountered. Peter used his time in prison to build what he called "The Inside Track," a collection of insights and strategies for thriving in challenging environments.

Since then, Peter has accomplished an impressive list of seemingly impossible feats, including most recently a row across the Atlantic ocean with one friend in a small boat.

Serena Williams: Physical, Mental, and Emotional Resilience

Serena Williams, one of the greatest athletes in the history of tennis, exemplifies how building a custom toolkit is about much more than physical ability--it's about mental and emotional resilience, adaptability, and the willingness to evolve. Throughout her career, Serena has faced countless challenges, both on and off the court, yet her ability to adapt and fine-tune her approach allowed her to dominate the world of tennis for over two decades.

From a young age, Serena learned the value of hard work and perseverance. Trained by her father on public courts in Compton, California, she and her sister Venus developed not only their technical skills but also an unshakable mindset of determination. As Serena's career progressed, she realized that success wasn't just about physical ability-- it was about continuously evolving her toolkit to include mental fortitude, emotional intelligence, and strategic adaptation.

Serena's career has been filled with comebacks, most notably her return to tennis after giving birth in 2017. Facing a life-threatening complication during childbirth, Serena was forced to confront her own physical limitations in ways she had never experienced before. But instead of letting this setback derail her career, she used it as an opportunity to expand her toolkit—focusing not only on her physical recovery but also on her mental and emotional resilience. She has since spoken openly about the mental challenges of motherhood, health struggles, and the pressures of being in the public eye, showing that her success stems not just from her talent, but from her ability to adapt and find inspiration in adversity.

Jay Samit: A Master of Disruption

I would be remiss if I did not mention Jay Samit after mentioning the power of disruption. His book Disrupt You!, was highly influential in my own journey of transformation, and since it has been translated into more than 10 languages, it is safe to say it has influenced countless others as well.

I had the pleasure of interviewing Jay briefly in early 2020 on my very own Authentic Action Podcast, just as the lockdowns began across this country. His early career includes several examples of bold disruption, and he generously shares his wisdom in talks and most recently also through his artwork. He teaches a method of success that involves looking for problems to solve and then finding unique and bold solutions that disrupt old patterns that are no longer functioning optimally.

During the pandemic he surprised me by diving into a passion I didn't even know he had, which is a delightful style of watercolor. He turned this into a series of paintings and then a book, which I am delighted to own a signed copy of. This is just another example of how he took a potential problem (being locked down during the pandemic) and turned it into a beautiful and creative solution (thought provoking 'pop art' that manages to make deep social commentary in a playful, colorful way).

Adapting, Evolving, and Building Unique Toolkits

The stories of Peter Sage, Serena Williams, and Jay Samit all demonstrate the power of building a custom toolkit--one that adapts to the challenges we face. Of course, these are just a few examples in a world filled with individuals who've forged their own paths by crafting personalized approaches to success.

Each of them reminds us that it's not about following someone else's blueprint but about figuring out what works for us, refining those tools, and then using them to reach new heights.

Take Tim Ferriss, for instance, whose unconventional approach to productivity has inspired millions to rethink how they work and live. In The 4-Hour Workweek, Ferriss offers a toolkit designed to streamline effort and focus on what truly matters--challenging the traditional idea that success requires constant grinding. He teaches that by hacking our own systems, we can accomplish more by doing less, showing us that sometimes, less is more. His methods are all about finding what works for you, rather than getting caught in the trap of doing things the way everyone else does them.

Another inspiration to many is Bruce Lee, whose philosophy wasn't just about martial arts--it was about life. Lee believed in taking from many different schools of thought, absorbing what was useful, discarding what wasn't, and adding what was uniquely his own. He reminds us that rigid adherence to one system can be limiting. Instead, it's about blending methods, being flexible, and creating a toolkit that's adaptable to the situation. His approach wasn't just about throwing punches, it was about building a mindset that could evolve with him, ready for any challenge.

Chloe Kim, a two-time Olympic gold medalist in snowboarding, is another powerful example of someone who has crafted her own path. Known for her daring tricks and fearless style, Kim faced enormous pressure from a young age to perform on the world stage.

After winning her first Olympic gold at just 17, she took a break to focus on her mental health and rediscover her love for the sport. She built a toolkit that wasn't just about physical training--it was about balancing ambition with self-care, knowing when to push forward and when to take a step back. Kim's story shows us that success isn't just about mastering one aspect of life: it's about evolving your mindset, managing pressure, and finding joy in the process.

Again, these are just a few examples among countless others--people who have learned to adapt, experiment, and build toolkits that work for them. Each of them teaches us that success doesn't come from following a set script. Instead, it's about figuring out what resonates, what fuels you, and what tools will help you navigate the unique challenges you face.

As you build your own toolkit, keep in mind that it's personal--it's yours. It's okay to take a bit from here, a bit from there, and leave behind what doesn't work. Learn from the stories of others, experiment with what fits, and create a toolkit that's as flexible and evolving as you are.

The Shift. Own your emotions; Own your life.

Because there's no one right way--there's only your way,
and that's exactly what makes it powerful and gives you
your power back.

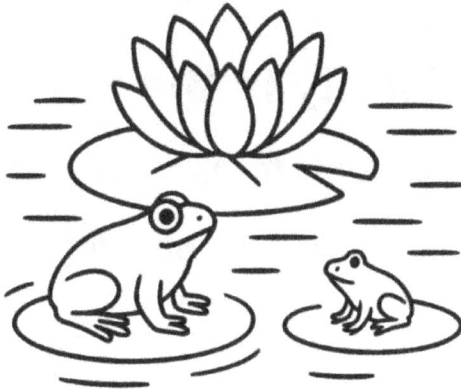

CHAPTER 6

Clarity in the Mud

Master your *emotions by labeling them*

Bringing Beautiful Things to the Surface

The Power of Naming Things

Remember, Feelings Are Not Facts, but they ARE information that your body wants you to know. By design, you only notice the emotions that rise above the regular 'hum', so they are going to tend to be the ones that 'set off' or trigger some 'alarm system' that tells you something needs your special attention.

Feelings are stories we tell about emotions, and they can be wonderful guidance to help you become more authentic, coherent, and vibrant. Once we realize the vast majority of stories our brains come up with are not entirely (or sometimes even partially) true, it becomes easy to see why it is so important to stop allowing those stories to 'run away' with our emotions. Some of us get stuck spinning our wheels for decades in trauma loops before we make the important choice to shift.

The Shift. Own your emotions; Own your life.

Congratulations for having the courage or at least the curiosity to explore the potentials that learning to re-regulate your emotions can have on your life! This really can be life-changing, and you can make significant changes by choosing even one tool.

Putting It All Together

Now that we have introduced the tools, let's start to put together just a few that work best for you. It's important to keep in mind the desired outcome for this entire process is for you to feel like you are running your own life, confidently and competently.

You have permission to pick and choose the tools that make the most sense for you and ignore the others, at least for now. Over time you are likely to find you may start to learn to use more of the tools in this book or find other tools which I did not include. This is all perfect!

Many of us are taught early in life that some emotions are good and some are bad. It is very common for humans to celebrate and 'drum up' more ecstasy and joy and suppress anger and sadness. However, any extreme emotion can be a signal that you are veering 'off course'. Perhaps a better way of thinking of it is that you might be slowing down your evolution by intensifying the swing of things.

Also, your system is designed to always aim at homeostasis, so having extreme positives can lead to extreme negatives. When we are criticizing someone else, that is a clue there is something in us that we are denying and ashamed of. When we put someone else on a pedestal and think they are better than us, that is a clue that there is something in us we want to cultivate or an invitation to look

263

more closely at our true desires and bring more of that into our conscious lives.

The recent influx of diagnosed 'disorders' including neurodivergence, autism, CPTSD, bipolar disorder, personality disorders, depression, anxiety, panic, and ADHD can all be viewed through the simple lens of a build-up and stagnation of unprocessed and unbalanced emotions.

By focusing on rebalancing polarity, rather than giving more momentum to the direction of the emotion, you can learn to rebalance your own mental and emotional state.

Your biological system simply wants homeostasis and wants to keep your consciousness and unconsciousness working together, moving in the same direction. The feeling of chaos and turbulence in your psyche is simply your guidance system trying to guide you back into alignment.

If you can shift from a story of 'defective' to a story of 'opportunity', you will be delighted at the positive changes you will see in your life, sometimes instantly.

I do think that those of us being labeled as neurodivergent rather than neurotypical (labels which are only helpful in certain contexts and sometimes do more harm than good) tend to be extra sensitive to these sensations, and also sometimes have a lack of capacity to process them, which can lead to a nervous system that is frequently or chronically in a dysregulated state.

It could take some extra time to develop new strategies and find the most effective tools if this describes you. Be patient and compassionate with yourself as you learn to do this. Keep a 'success journal' or 'good feeling jar' that you can draw from when you need extra confidence or a moral boost.

Do you believe the stories you tell yourself about your emotions? Do you interpret them as accurate messages that require logical responses, or are they chaotic and messy and hard to understand?

Many of us have had little or no training on how to interpret or handle our emotions. If you come from a family like mine, then you may have been encouraged to express some of your emotions and forbidden to express others.

Many of us have been shunned and shamed for having emotions or feelings at all. Negative and high-energy emotions are often discouraged or condemned in families and schools, while still being actively expressed in all sorts of unhealthy ways, and so at best we learn to use anger as fuel, sadness as justification, and joy as a reason to feel shameful.

Understanding and naming our emotions is a powerful tool for emotional mastery. When we accurately identify and label our feelings, we create the space needed to process them and allow them to settle, reducing their intensity and giving us greater control over our emotional states. Research in psychology and neuroscience supports this approach, showing that naming and processing emotions leads to better emotional regulation, reduced stress, and greater mental clarity.

Labeling Your Emotions

A key concept in emotional regulation is affect labeling, which refers to the act of naming an emotional experience.

The Shift. Own your emotions; Own your life.

Research published in Psychological Science demonstrated that naming emotions—such as saying, "I feel anxious" or "I'm angry"—can reduce the amygdala's activity, which is the brain's emotional center responsible for triggering stress and fear responses.

In the study, participants who labeled their emotions showed reduced emotional reactivity and greater activation in the prefrontal cortex, the part of the brain involved in decision-making and self-control. This shift helps us approach our emotions with greater clarity, reducing their intensity and giving us more control over how we respond.

Naming our emotions is like shining a light on a dark, unknown space. Instead of being overwhelmed by a vague emotional storm, we identify the specific feelings we are experiencing. This practice of affect labeling allows us to engage with our emotions in a more mindful, controlled way, rather than being swept away by them.

Processing Emotions: Letting Them Flow

While naming emotions is the first step, processing them is also essential for emotional mastery. Allowing ourselves to feel emotions and letting them move through us is a critical part of emotional regulation.

A study published in 2015 found that individuals who acknowledged and accepted their emotions experienced fewer negative emotional effects over time compared to those who tried to suppress or avoid their feelings.

Emotional suppression--trying to push emotions away-- tends to increase stress and leads to emotional dysregulation. In contrast, accepting and processing

266

emotions reduces their impact and helps them settle more quickly.

This finding aligns with the idea that emotions, when fully experienced and allowed to flow, tend to self-regulate. Instead of trying to fight or avoid them, we can reduce emotional buildup by giving our feelings space to be felt. This approach also fosters emotional resilience, as we become more comfortable with the ebb and flow of our emotions without needing to escape them.

Allowing Emotions to Settle

When we give ourselves time and space to acknowledge, process, and let emotions calm down, we create room for more rational decision-making. Mindfulness practices, which encourage non-judgmental awareness of emotions, help people experience emotions fully without becoming overwhelmed by them. This leads to improved emotional clarity and better emotional regulation over time.

By allowing emotions to settle, we're able to gain perspective and respond to situations from a place of balance rather than emotional reactivity. This moment of pause--where we let emotions flow, settle, and process naturally--gives us the opportunity to approach life's challenges with a clearer, more grounded mindset.

The research is clear: naming, processing, and allowing emotions to settle not only helps reduce the intensity of our feelings but also enhances emotional regulation and fosters long-term emotional mastery. These tools empower us to face emotions head-on, rather than letting them control our behaviors or decisions.

The Shift. Own your emotions; Own your life.

One tool I have found very helpful for processing emotions that feel 'mixed up', unclear, or overwhelming is doodling. For nearly a year during one of my most challenging times of perimenopause, doodling became a way for me to play with very heavy and dark emotions.

During that time, I created a journal of cartoon doodles with two penguin characters to represent masculine and feminine aspects in my personal relationships. I eventually created several other characters as well, and for many months I used this practice to help untangle and give voice to my mixed-up feelings.

Making them into crude characters and allowing myself the freedom to express difficult emotions through the characters I created was profoundly healing. The end result is a crass series that makes me smile when I reflect on one of the most difficult periods of my life.

The Struggle Is Real...but it's also made up.

Those of us who were severely abused or neglected by our primary caregivers or siblings may have learned to unconsciously suppress our natural defenses in order to survive. This often leads to a continuation of the abusive pattern because it is an unconscious coping mechanism.

I have watched many families struggle with the effects of this unconscious playing out of defensiveness in unhealthy ways. If you cannot say "no" or "stop that" without experiencing an escalation, you might have internalized that feeling and it could become self-destructive.

I believe this was a major factor in my own history of autoimmunity. My body started to turn against itself and attack my own tissues when it became highly activated with no healthy ways to process my feelings or no outlet for expressing the deep sense of defensiveness that I felt in response to having my body and safety threatened repeatedly in infancy and early childhood.

Of course, there are other lenses to view this through. Natural hormones and pharmaceutical hormones like birth control and many other chemicals can play a significant role in how our immune system, and other bodily systems, function. There are multiple external and internal factors and again, most of them are out of our control, but some of them are more in our control than we might like to think.

Our current industrial disease complex can be especially harmful to female systems, for numerous reasons, and in numerous ways.

Females and males are often raised with very different programming and expectations, on top of our natural physical, hormonal and other differences. It is worth mentioning that if you have been programmed to believe that your worth is wrapped up in overriding your own needs and desires to care for others because of your gender (or any other aspect of your identity), as is the case for a majority of women and many men, then it may take extra work to really get to the root of your core values and navigate life with fewer feelings of resentment or disempowerment.

It is my desire to offer a fresh perspective of the potential value of all our emotions, while also encouraging us to put them in a different context when it comes to how we think about our emotional responses.

Relying too heavily on emotions without reason is just as foolish as relying too heavily on reason without intuition or feelings. Both of these can be associated with the two hemispheres of the brain.

In his epic, ground-breaking book, *The Master and His Emissary,* Ian McGilchrist explores how we need these two aspects to work together to really get a full picture of reality and be able to function at our fullest capacity.

It is only when something 'trips a wire' of being outside our own personal 'normal' that we even notice a change.

This is how divers who train to over-ride the anxiety of carbon dioxide poisoning can end up dying instantaneously. They learn to override and ignore their body's natural signals that something is wrong until eventually their body stops signaling. We are incredibly adaptable beings which also makes us highly trainable, or easy to program. I urge you to take an active, participatory interest in your own programming.

The Shift. Own your emotions; Own your life.

Your body does the best it can to alert you to danger, but if you don't take the time to get to know yourself in a loving, curious way, or if you train your body that you do not listen to it, it may find new ways of letting you know things are not okay.

That might sound obvious to you, or you might find you have some resistance to this idea, so let's break it down a bit more.

Our emotions and feelings are indeed messages from our bodies, the result of chemical cascades that happen in response to data received and transferred to various parts of body systems or the whole body.

I am not saying we should disregard our emotions or feelings or act like they are not happening. I am saying that our interpretations of our emotions, what we call our feelings, are often underdeveloped and so misinterpreted, or interpreted in unhelpful, often very unhealthy ways.

If you do not take time to understand what your emotions are communicating and respond with what your body needs, you are likely to end up feeling like a slave to your own emotions.

Learning to listen to the feelings we have can be an excellent way to start to learn how to give ourselves what we need and get to the root of our true desires. We can get to know ourselves and come to a better understanding of our interpretations of the chemical responses that are created in response to what is going on around and inside us.

It's important to realize, however, that the stories we tell ourselves about the emotional responses we have are often rooted in misinterpretations, false programs, unresolved conflicts, and traumas.

Currently, I see many people who either suppress and ignore most of their emotions, distract ourselves from them or dive deeply into them without reservation, and react as if our interpretations of our own emotions, or our feelings, are facts, rather than clues, or data to be put into a larger equation or picture.

Simply shutting down or turning off your emotions is not an effective long-term strategy for success.

I am pretty far
from okay.

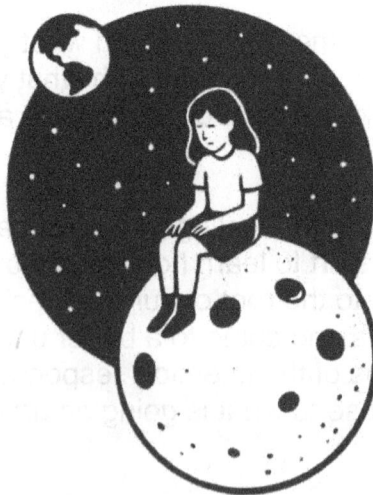

The Shift. Own your emotions; Own your life.

If you simply learn to ignore or shut down in response to having emotions, as many seemingly successful people do, you could end up being one of the beings who is hurting everyone around you without understanding why. Eventually people can become so unfeeling that they don't even notice or care when they hurt others.

Your feelings are messages you can use, and simply ignoring them or shutting them down will not make the messages irrelevant. It will simply make you unaware of them. Most of us don't want to be a person who hurts others, and yet, we often do ignore our feelings to the point that we ignore other people's feelings too.

If you have a reoccurring pattern of people around you accusing you of being insensitive, there is probably some truth in that which could be useful to examine. At the same time, we can only be responsible for our own feelings. Other people's feelings are not our responsibility.

Imagine there is a car alarm going off outside. It only makes sense to ignore the alarm or turn it off AFTER you have evaluated the situation to see what set the alarm off. If you have an alarm that starts going off all the time when it shouldn't, then it needs repairing or replacing.

Your nervous system is similar to the car alarm in this analogy. It is there to help you, and if it seems like 'a bother' then take a little time to figure out why. Simply ignoring it or unplugging it does not fix whatever the issue is.

If other people's emotions are upsetting to you, and you find yourself shutting down, blocking them out, or humiliating them for being emotional, consider that you could be part of their problem.

The Shift. Own your emotions; Own your life.

Even if you think you have your emotions 'under control', they are still driving you and influencing the other humans around you. It is worth examining them even if you believe it isn't.

It always 'takes two to tango'--two people to meet anywhere-- and your conflicts are never 'just the other person'. If they were, you wouldn't be aware of them.

Women, especially, are equipped with intuitive senses that many men are not as in touch with. There are of course nuances and variations in all categories, but this is generally true in humans.

The current paradigm shuns women as 'emotional' and shuns men as weak if they show emotions. This ultimately hurts us all. Hysteria was a documentable disorder in the great made-up manual of disorders up until 1980, and our current society still treats women with incredible disrespect and disregard for our health and safety. Hormonal fluctuations play a significant role in our emotions and our feelings, or the stories we tell ourselves about what we notice in ourselves.

If you have a woman in your life, especially if that woman is you, please keep this in mind. Hold a safe space for her and learn what intuition can do. Women have honed the ability to feel feelings and recognize intuitive impulses over generations to be able to care for infants and raise children.

Rather than shutting down, narrowing your perspective on emotions and labeling them as simply 'good' or 'bad', try shifting your perspective. See if you can find a more nuanced label for how you are feeling. If your feeling was a cartoon character, what would it look like? What would it say? How would it behave? What would it need?

The Shift. Own your emotions; Own your life.

Get curious and ask yourself 'what is my body trying to communicate to me, really?' A good place to start is to notice where you feel it in your body, and what it feels like. Practice naming and being curious.

Please note, this has not come easily for me, and it is natural and normal for it to take a good deal of practice.

Another tool that has been helpful for me when dealing with intense feelings is to write 'on behalf of' a particular part or aspect of myself that I am struggling with. This could be an aspect, such as my 'child self' or the 'rebellious teen" side of myself; or it could be a specific body part, like my spleen, tooth, or the pain in my arms. I would start by writing or saying something like:

"Dear wounded child aspect, I am here to see you, and to love you. Please tell me what you want me to know, and how I can help you to feel better."

Then I would write freely, pretending to write as that aspect. Sometimes I would use a special pen or allow my handwriting to take on a particular style. There are no hard and fast rules to this type of work, except to listen to yourself and practice being compassionate. This type of exercise can be profoundly revealing and deeply healing.

What research and science has found so far:

One thing that has been studied regarding emotions and feelings, is what we call them. Research has shown that most of us have only a few words to describe the complex myriads of emotions our bodies are capable of. Glad, sad, and mad are the most common states which people in my culture can identify.

275

The Shift. Own your emotions; Own your life.

Many of us use only a few words to describe our emotions. Research shows that as we begin to expand our vocabulary about them, we also expand our ability to handle them in healthy ways.

There is also good research to show that the more specific we can get about describing our emotions to ourselves, the more useful they can become.

For example, rather than just thinking "I am sad, or mad, or angry", if we can get curious about it, add a pause, and dive a bit deeper, we will often discover an unarticulated desire or boundary under our emotions. If we can become more aware of the specific, more nuanced boundaries and desires that our emotions are responding to; then our emotions and the feelings become messengers, clues, and helpful guides, rather than hindrances and disruptions to be quelled and calmed.

Keep in mind that the point is not to label them and make them part of our identity or impose them on others as their identity. It is important not to 'mistake the finger for the moon'. Naming things does not fully define them. It simply helps us gain a greater sense of control as we allow them to move through us, and often allows them to dissipate or lose strength more quickly.

The naming of our emotions does not fully describe or express them. The objective of naming them is to help you rebalance them, make more sense of them, and to help you gain some sense of control over them. Hopefully you will also start to recognize the fueling and guiding potential they hold.

Much like labeling boxes in a garage or closet, it can be helpful to label our emotions accurately and to explore, document, and take inventory of them somewhat regularly.

The Shift. Own your emotions; Own your life.

This way we can make sure we keep our thoughts, beliefs, and actions in line with our values.

Nearly all dis-ease can be viewed through this lens of alignment and coherence, and it is not hard to see that incongruence and incoherence interfere with the body's natural ability to heal. Internal and external clutter interferes with healing and with living a fully functional life.

When we have very high-energy emotions, they often 'stir up' lots of sentiments and sediments which can literally cloud our judgment. There are several studies that indicate that negative emotions like anger may rev themselves up when we express them, rather than dissipate. They can also become toxic if stuffed down into the body and not processed.

It is important to learn to 'take your foot off the gas' when emotions are high, pause, and take some time to untangle them and let the intensity settle before making choices and taking action to remedy them.

The long-standing "count to ten" advice when we are angry or upset is a good place to start as it can help create the necessary pause to then make a different choice. If you can add a nice long exhale and a mental reframing, then you will have successfully navigated a challenging emotional situation or neuro-chemical cascade.

This is a great strategy when dealing with our modern-day tendencies to be overstimulated and over-reactionary. Obviously, in real emergencies, when we need to fight or flee or freeze (or fawn), this tendency to switch into the sympathetic nervous system and override our prefrontal cortex, or higher reasoning system is also worth 'tuning up' so that it functions to help us navigate these situations in the best ways possible. Left undisciplined and unexamined, this system often functions poorly at best, and malfunctions often. Panic is almost never the most productive solution.

Zoom in-Zoom out

It can be helpful to narrow or expand your focus on a situation to help you gain a better understanding. Imagine if you were someone passing by right now. How would you describe yourself? Now imagine you are a tiny investigator measuring the molecules of your neurochemistry and guessing what emotion you are about to be feeling. What is your prediction?

Shifting your perspective is an easy way to change the story of how things are, and by doing that, you can change the way you feel.

Sometimes it is helpful to get more specific about naming our emotions, and other times it can be helpful to break it down to a more binary view. On a fundamental level, all emotions are either expansive or contracting; and can be seen as love or fear.

I like to say that fear is just love underinformed, for if you really dig underneath what you fear, you are likely to find something you love.

For example, maybe you realize you are angry when you scream at a stranger who cuts it a little too close for comfort in traffic. Maybe you feel a sudden flash of anger and think "Dumbass is gonna kill somebody", or maybe even something more intense.

After the initial chemical hit from that flash of anger, you might feel a tinge of resistance as you struggle internally

The Shift. Own your emotions; Own your life.

back and forth between a sense of shame for not controlling your anger and a sense of indignation and justification, perpetuating a chemical cycle which could be controlling many aspects of your life.

One way you might find helpful to break the cycle is to notice and name the emotion more specifically. For example, maybe at first you think 'that guy really pissed me off…if I hadn't slammed on the brakes, I might have rear-ended him and cost us both…"

If you think about what is underneath feeling pissed off at the other driver, you are likely to find another stressor underneath the initial flash of anger. Maybe you are worried about finances and ultimately stressed about not taking good care of your health. Maybe you are feeling unfulfilled at work. Maybe you are feeling insecure about an intimate relationship. Maybe you just spent a lot of money on your vehicle. Whatever the reason for your feelings, the flavor and intensity is going to have more to do with you than with the other driver, and how you respond is going to impact your future.

Whatever the underlying emotions are, you might have better luck processing them when you can own them and get more specific about what they are. You might also get good results from going more meta, or broad, and boiling your emotions down to a binary love or fear quality. Then see if you can recognize what is it you love or what is it you really fear (and can you trace that fear back farther to some love)?

INVITATION TO ACTION: Imagine you are a little bird in the windowsill of the room or place you are in,

The Shift. Own your emotions; Own your life.

or a fly on the wall. Picture yourself from that distance, right now. What would you guess is going on inside you, if you were looking at you from the outside. Do the inside and outside match? Why or why not?

This perspective shift practice is helpful anytime you notice yourself telling a story you don't like about any situation or circumstance. If you don't like the look of things, try shifting your perspective and look at it another way.

What is normal?

What happens to you has an effect. If this system becomes over-activated it can begin to malfunction frequently, and then we call that PTSD or an anxiety or panic disorder, or another psychological malfunction. However, in my experience, the mental aspect of this, the story we tell ourselves about what is happening, is secondary to the chemical reactions in the body, or the emotional responses, are often misaligned with what is going on and with the responses we want to have.

To my perception, this is a major factor that has led to our current state of rising suicide rates and increasing psychological dysfunction. This has gotten so extreme over the last decade or so that society seems increasingly in danger of being destroyed by our inability to think clearly and make coherent choices.

While I agree that this is not a highly functional or desirable state, I don't think it is helpful to view it as abnormal or a disease or "syndrome". The work of Gabor Mate, Zack Bush, Joe Dispenza, Michael Pollan, Bruce Lipton, and

The Shift. Own your emotions; Own your life.

many others in the last decade helps to bring a much different perspective into focus.

The idea that there is some 'normal' that we should be aiming for is absurd and falls apart when you really get into real-life situations. I find the idea of coherence, and settling, much more useful.

As highlighted in many popular books such as Oprah's book, What Happened to You? and Bessel Vander Kolk's book, The Body Keeps the Score, the traumas we endure end up making a mark not just in our stories and emotional bodies but in our physical bodies as well. This is true of traumas that are both subtle and complex, like emotional abuse or neglect, and those that are more significant and straightforward, like a car accident or a tsunami.

Trauma settles into our bodies and into our story lines when we don't take time to grieve, process, and ultimately shake things off.

It can feel like a "catch-22" when it comes to being honest about our experiences and emotions, not living in denial, and not defining ourselves by our past traumas and perpetuate our limiting beliefs.

When we define ourselves as defective or disordered and start to identify as that, as if everything is not temporary, we often hold ourselves in that state longer than we would if we simply examined our state and then started to take necessary actions to bring ourselves back to that calmer center lane before we make choices or take actions. **It's important to balance the acceptance of limitations with the relentless knowing that the seemingly impossible and obviously improbable is absolutely, completely possible.**

281

The Shift. Own your emotions; Own your life.

A useful technique when struggling with limiting beliefs or self-defeating thoughts on repeat is to add the words "right now", "so far" or "yet" to the end of a limiting statement. These are magic words which open spaces of possibility for change. I encourage you to use them often.

Many of my personal and professional relationships have been damaged by my lack of understanding of this. I see people around me every day who are wounding one another, often the people they love the most, because of what seems to be a lack of understanding of this basic idea.

When we label each other or ourselves as damaged or defective without adding a sense that it is a temporary state that we can remedy, we are creating more incoherence and incongruity in our lives and that permeates society.

As I mentioned, there are times in life when we do want this system to be in the driver's seat. We are capable of incredible feats, such as lifting a car off a child, running incredibly far or fast, or enduring unimaginable pain in order to survive or help someone we care about survive. This system is a beautiful mechanism that serves us well in some situations.

However, in our modern society, we are often bombarded with activating and triggering sights, sounds, smells, and ideas. If we do not consciously take steps to manage this in healthy ways, we are likely to get bounced and drug around by this overstimulating, stirring up and eventually sort of 'burning out' of our limbic system. This is why developing a regular practice of remaining or returning to a more calm and coherent state is crucial to building a fulfilling and vibrant life.

The Shift. Own your emotions; Own your life.

"Peace is the result of retraining your mind to process life as it is, rather than how you think it should be." Wayne Dyer

Learning to Let Emotions Settle: Finding Clarity in the Mud

When life feels chaotic, it can be easy to confuse movement with progress. The question is: are you settling or simmering? Are you stirring things up at just the right moments for growth, or are you constantly creating turbulence in your emotional waters? Finding clarity often means learning when to let things settle—like allowing muddy water to become still until you can see clearly again.

Much like the lotus flower that rises from the mud, your growth and self-mastery can emerge from the murk of emotional turmoil, but only if you give the sediment time to settle.

The lotus grows in muddy waters, yet it blooms pure and unblemished above the surface. In the same way, we must learn to navigate the 'mud' of our emotions and life's challenges. It is in this muddy water--our discomfort, uncertainty, and emotional chaos--that we find the nutrients for growth. But first, we must allow the mud to settle to see the path forward.

Are you keeping a healthy, dynamic balance in all the major areas of your life, or are there certain areas that feel stuck in the mud? Do you manage both the highs and the lows with equal coherence, or do you find yourself self-sabotaging more during one than the other?

Sometimes, we may become more prone to sabotage when we're at a high point, letting excitement or success cloud our judgment. Other times, we sink into the mud

The Shift. Own your emotions; Own your life.

during our low moments, unsure of how to pull ourselves back up.

The key is learning to "settle the sediment" to let the turbulence within calm before you re-engage with life or pursue your goals.

This is an ongoing habit, a practice you must cultivate regularly. It's helpful to think of your emotional regulation tools in the context of red, yellow, and green light tools. Depending on the severity of your emotional state, you can use the appropriate tool to bring yourself back into balance.

Daily meditation practice is one of the most proven and accessible ways to allow your internal mud to settle. By sitting in stillness—noticing, breathing, allowing, practicing gratitude if you can--even for just a few minutes each day, you create space for clarity to emerge. It's available to everyone, no matter what their circumstances.

Even in the most extreme situations--like Nelson Mandela's, when he kept his faith in the human capacity for peace throughout decades in prison, you can create a safe haven in your mind. Meditation helps you cultivate coherence in your body and mind, allowing you to return to your goals and life decisions with renewed clarity.

I also find sound healing or chanting practices to be highly effective. Vibrations we produce when we hum or sing, stimulate our vagus nerve and activate the parasympathetic nervous system. This can help switch us back to a calmer, less dysregulated state in just a couple minutes.

I find a regular practice of 5-15 minutes of sound healing every day is a great 'green light' tool. It makes me feel much more regulated throughout the rest of the day. I also use this as a red or yellow light tool sometimes and find it highly effective to help calm me down or keep me calmer in stressful situations too.

Letting your emotions settle is more than just emotional regulation or resetting the nervous system. It's also about building resilience and strength, so you maintain a state of calm more often, even in the face of life's inevitable challenges. It's much like the difference between treating an acute injury and building overall strength, flexibility, and resilience over time. The tools and techniques you use may be similar, but the intention and approach will vary depending on the situation.

Remember, the goal is not perfection. Like the lotus, you are growing through the mud, and that growth comes with moments of messiness and uncertainty. But it is precisely from that mess that beauty and clarity can emerge.

Becoming Curious About Your Emotional Responses

When we become aware of an emotional response, it's a signal from our body that something needs our attention. Emotions arise when our internal system perceives a potential threat, an unmet need, or even a move closer or farther from a goal.

These emotional signals can be broad at first--good or bad, happy or sad--but part of mastering your emotions and developing emotional fitness is learning to dive deeper and become more curious about what your body is really trying to tell you.

The Shift. Own your emotions; Own your life.

Think of emotions like containers labeled with general terms. Initially, you might notice anger, frustration, or fear, but these are often surface-level emotions that contain something deeper. For example, under anger, you might find fear.

If you're frustrated because you can't figure something out, the underlying fear might be the fear of failure or uncertainty. These subtleties are crucial to understand because they give you more precise information about what's truly happening within you.

Start developing this skill by paying closer attention to your emotional responses. Whenever you notice an emotion surfacing, try adding another layer of description.

What are you *really* feeling? Physically I mean. Where in your body do you feel it? Is it a tightness in your chest, a burning in your stomach, or a contraction in your muscles?

As you tune in to these sensations, try not to fuel the discomfort, but instead use your awareness to shift your perspective and create a sense of organization within your emotional system.

The more nuanced your emotional vocabulary becomes, the more empowered you will be to harness the untapped potential within your body.

When you can label your emotions more precisely and start to recognize what sensations are registering in your body when you feel them, they become easier to process and put into perspective. You can start to unravel those tangled up messes of unprocessed emotions that you don't understand. You can determine what requires immediate attention and what can be addressed later, once the emotional mud has settled.

The Hidden Dysregulation in Positive Emotions

It's important to recognize that even positive emotions can be a sign of dysregulation. Up until relatively recently, I used to think only negative feelings indicated an imbalance in my system. But through experience, I've learned that even extreme highs can pull us out of alignment.

That "high", or elated feeling--whether it's from excitement, success, or any other positive event--can sometimes lead to poor decision-making or self-sabotage if we're not careful. Like Icarus, playing in the ocean waves and then flying too close to the sun, we can get carried away and make catastrophic errors when we are overly excited.

Even when our positive feelings are from being in an extremely productive flow state, that is probably not the best time to set new goals or make any big decisions about future plans or relationships. It is a good time to engage and enjoy the present moment fully.

Much like we manage the lows, we must also learn to manage the highs. It's about maintaining coherence and balance, regardless of where you are on the emotional spectrum. Whether you're riding a high or sinking into a low, the practice of letting your emotions settle and aiming towards more balance in your center will help you make more grounded, wise decisions as you navigate life's challenges.

The Shift. Own your emotions; Own your life.

Focus on Strengths, Not Just Weaknesses

The *80/20 principle*, also known as the Pareto Principle, is a concept that shows up in many aspects of life: 80% of outcomes come from 20% of efforts. This idea can be applied to your emotional landscape as well. Find those habits or aspects of your life that are having the greatest impact on your outcomes and make sure they are aligned with the person you want to be.

You can also use this guideline to make sure you are not paying too much attention to the negative aspects of your life. It's natural and normal to have some negative thoughts and feelings--after all, emotions are our body's way of signaling what needs attention. But if you find that the balance of negative thoughts is tipping beyond 10-20%, it might be time to adjust your focus.

It's not productive to spend much of your mental bandwidth trying to overcome every weakness or hurdle. Doing so can leave you feeling stuck in an endless cycle of self-improvement without ever enjoying the progress you've made.

Instead, apply the 80/20 principle to your emotional and mental energy: focus 80% of your attention on your strengths, the positives in your life, and the things that are going well. The remaining 20% can be used to acknowledge and address challenges, but don't let that 20% dominate your mindset. At the same time, find those aspects that seem small but have the greatest impact to help you improve your emotional fitness and thereby improve your overall life.

Shifting your focus in this way helps you harness the power of positivity. When you intentionally look for the things that are working, you build momentum and create a reinforcing cycle of growth.

By celebrating both your small and big wins, you give your mind and body the reinforcement they need to keep progressing. Success, no matter how small, builds confidence and strengthens your resilience.

It's important to remember that dwelling too much on what's not working can amplify those negative aspects and pull you further into a dysregulated state. Unfortunately, many of us have unknowingly practiced this by default. Try to balance out your natural tendency to focus on problems by developing practices that give equal or greater attention to your strengths and victories.

In practical terms, this might mean setting aside time each day to reflect on your successes--whether it's a small win like sticking to a healthy habit or a larger victory like achieving a long-term goal. By making this practice a habit, you condition your mind to focus on positive outcomes rather than getting bogged down by obstacles.

This doesn't mean ignoring your weaknesses or challenges but rather recognizing that focusing too much on them can drain your energy and cloud your vision. By maintaining a healthy balance--keeping negative thoughts in check while celebrating your strengths—you can keep moving forward with greater clarity and coherence.

The Shift. Own your emotions; Own your life.

Identifying Triggers

As you develop more awareness of your own emotions and start to see the patterns that have been governing so much of the story of your life, you will notice specific situations, people, stories, and even perhaps smells, colors or other things that trigger stronger emotional reactions in you. This is natural, and we all have them. Some will be nearly universal, or very common (such as feeling unworthy of love or like we are not enough), and some will be unique to you. Some of them will probably make easy sense, and others may be bewildering.

Identifying and untangling triggers can be a long and arduous process, so it is important to pace yourself. It's also important to know that you do not need to identify or dissolve all (or even most) or your triggers to heal. You can develop more Emotional Fitness and become less reactive, regardless of what your triggers are.

Especially at first, it is enough to begin to notice what types of things inspire you with specific types of internal stories. You do NOT have to untangle them to practice your emotional regulation tools and develop more emotional fitness. Over time the triggers will have less control over you even if you never untangle any of them, and many will also unravel themselves if you just leave them alone for a while.

Emotional Dysregulation and Its Connection to Currently Common and Significant Disorders

There are many officially labeled disorders that are associated with emotional regulation, often to a more extreme and sometimes debilitating degree. These include autism spectrum disorder (ASD), attention-deficit/hyperactivity disorder (ADHD), borderline personality disorder (BPD), anxiety disorders, depression, post-traumatic stress disorder (PTSD), and substance use disorders.

It's important to understand that these labels do not dictate the level of dysregulation and subsequent disfunction a person will experience. Rather, these labels are often a result of having frequent dysregulation and disfunction. Emotional fitness is a key factor in our mental and physical wellbeing.

If you suffer with one (or more) of these more challenging disorders, it is important to understand that there are different reasons we become dysregulated and when we know what that reason is, we have a much better chance of giving ourselves what we need to get back on track.

For example, people with autism may suffer from sensory overload and need to reduce stimulation to avoid a meltdown or reset after dysregulation, whereas people with ADHD may need something more stimulating like exercise or rhythmic music to help bring them into a more coherent state. Finding the right tools gets a lot easier when we start to understand more about our own patterns, habits, and underlying beliefs.

The Shift. Own your emotions; Own your life.

Self-Compassion and Grace

Please be gentle with yourself as you go through this healing process, especially in those times when you feel frustrated or unsupported.

There will be times that others let you down or that you feel betrayed or abandoned by important people or systems in your life. This is simply a part of life, but it still stings sometimes, and it is natural to feel disappointed and sad and frustrated sometimes. Give yourself some Grace. It's okay.

If you choose to accept that challenging and unpleasant feelings will arise sometimes and allow them to arrive and pass in their own time, you will be able to appreciate that even these more difficult feelings help give our lives meaning, and all of them are temporary.

"Normality is a paved road: it's comfortable to walk, but no flowers grow on it." ~ Vincent van Gogh

The Shift. Own your emotions; Own your life.

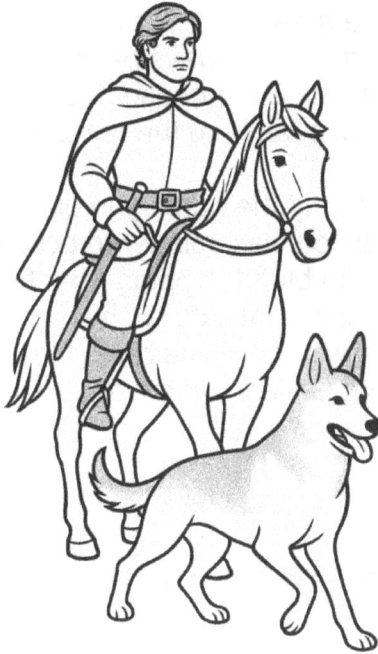

The Legend of Gellert the Faithful Dog

Once upon a time, in the kingdom of Gwynedd in North
Wales, there lived a noble and kind-hearted prince named
Llewelyn. He was known for his bravery in battle and his
wisdom as a ruler. Prince Llewelyn had many treasures,
but none more valuable to him than his faithful dog, Gellert.
Gellert was a large and loyal German Shepherd, who had
accompanied the prince on countless hunts and protected
him from many dangers.

One day, the prince decided to go hunting in the
mountains. Before leaving, he kissed his infant son
goodbye and entrusted the boy's safety to his most faithful
companion, Gellert. Confident that his son was in safe
hands, Llewelyn set off with his men.

293

The Shift. Own your emotions; Own your life.

When the prince returned home after the hunt, he was surprised not to be greeted by Gellert at the gate. This was unusual, as Gellert would always be the first to welcome him home. With a sense of unease, Llewelyn hurried into the castle and went straight to the nursery.

To his horror, he found the nursery in disarray. The cradle was overturned, blood was splattered across the floor, and Gellert stood by with blood dripping from his mouth. The prince looked around frantically for his son but saw no sign of him. Overcome with grief and rage, Llewelyn jumped to the conclusion that Gellert had savagely killed his beloved child.

Without a second thought, Llewelyn drew his sword and, in a fit of anguish, plunged it into Gellert's heart. The loyal dog let out a final, pained yelp and collapsed at his master's feet.

As Gellert's dying cry echoed through the castle, Llewelyn heard the sound of a baby crying. He frantically searched the room and soon discovered his son, unharmed, hidden beneath the overturned cradle. Nearby, the prince saw the lifeless body of a huge wolf. It was then that the terrible truth dawned on him: Gellert had not killed his son; he had saved the child from a ferocious wolf that had crept into the nursery. The blood on the dog's mouth was not his son's, but the wolf's.

Grief-stricken and filled with remorse, Llewelyn realized the grave mistake he had made. He had killed his most loyal and faithful friend, the one who had protected his son at the cost of his own life. Overcome with sorrow, Llewelyn buried Gellert with great honor and built a cairn over his grave.

From that day forward, the prince never smiled again. He could not forgive himself for acting in haste and killing the

The Shift. Own your emotions; Own your life.

faithful hound who had saved his son. The town where Gellert was buried is said to be named Beddgelert, which means "Gellert's Grave," in memory of the brave and loyal dog.

INVITATION TO ACTION: Think about a time in your life when emotional dysregulation caused you to act in a way that you later regrated. Maybe you hurt someone you love. Maybe you abandoned yourself or put yourself in a dangerous situation.

Now reflect on how your life and relationships might be better if you learn to recognize when you are dysregulated and 'take your foot off the gas' or pause, question, breathe, and re-regulate before moving forward.

Summary of Chapter Six

Emotions are like a special language that your body speaks, and our feelings are the stories we tell ourselves about the sensations we notice in response to them. Practice naming them more specifically, and also, loosen your grip a little bit when it comes to interpreting your feelings. There is often more going on in and around you than you are consciously aware of. Give yourself and those around you a little extra space and grace whenever you can.

Simply noticing and acknowledging when you are feeling overwhelmed and depressed is a good first step. The next step is to accept that this is a normal, natural reaction to your circumstances and treat yourself with compassion and patience rather than using recognition as fuel to add more negative energy to the situation.

As you practice loving yourself unconditionally, becoming the parent that your wounded inner child needs, you will find it gets easier to decide to get curious and find out why. Let the turbulence of emotional dysregulation settle before making important decisions!

Learning to take responsibility for changing the course of your life does not always come easily, as a single shift, but rather, as yet another series of shifts. Without the correct tools, sometimes diving deeper into your emotions simply leads to more and more dysregulation.

Make a regular habit of pausing and shifting so you can bring subtle and significant changes that will permeate every aspect of your life. Again and again, keep refining your perspective and uncovering things the things you do not want to look at. Deal with things you have been putting off by avoiding those negative feelings. Take a good, hard, honest look at yourself, but gently now, with compassion and patience.

Real People Who Inspire Me:

Nick Vujicic: Defying Limits and Inspiring the World

Nick Vujicic's story is one of extreme physical challenges transformed into a source of global inspiration. Born without arms or legs due to a rare disorder called Tetra-amelia syndrome, Nick faced overwhelming difficulties from birth. As a child, he struggled with depression, bullying, and the deep emotional pain of feeling "different." At just 10 years old, Nick attempted suicide, convinced that his life would never hold meaning.

It was in these darkest moments that Nick found his inner strength. He discovered that his worth wasn't defined by his physical limitations but by his ability to inspire and empower others. He took control of his narrative, refusing to be defined by what he lacked and instead focusing on what he could give.

Nick became a motivational speaker, traveling the world to share his message of hope, self-love, and perseverance. Like the lotus rising from the mud, his disabilities became the very foundation of his life's purpose--to show others that they, too, can rise from their darkest moments.

Nick's story is a powerful reminder that what might seem like a disadvantage can often be a unique gift. By embracing his challenges, Nick transformed his life into one of profound impact, reminding us that the mud of our struggles can help us bloom in ways we never imagined.

Jim Kwik: Rewriting the Script on Learning and the Brain

Jim Kwik's early life was marked by a traumatic brain injury that severely impacted his ability to learn. As a young child, Kwik was labeled "the boy with the broken brain" after a head injury left him with severe learning disabilities. Struggling to keep up in school, Kwik often felt defeated and isolated, believing that he would never amount to much. The constant frustration of feeling "less than" created a deep well of pain and self-doubt, much like the muddy waters from which the lotus must rise.

Jim refused to accept that narrative. Inspired and motivated by a mentor who believed in him, he began to teach himself how to learn, experimenting with different techniques and eventually developing methods to improve memory, focus, and brain function. Kwik's setbacks became the driving force behind his later success--he turned his learning disabilities into a superpower, developing brain-training programs used by people around the world. He took control of his narrative, reshaping his identity from "broken" to "brilliant."

Temple Grandin: Harnessing Difference as Strength

Diagnosed with autism at a time when the condition was even more poorly understood, and rarely diagnosed in girls, Temple Grandin faced significant societal and personal challenges. As a child, she struggled with communication, sensory overload, and the feeling of being an outsider. These aspects--her difference and the world's misunderstanding of it--could have easily left her isolated and unfulfilled.

Instead, Temple embraced her unique perspective, using it as a tool to revolutionize the livestock industry with more humane practices. Her deep empathy for animals and her ability to think visually allowed her to solve problems in ways others could not.

By integrating the shadow of societal rejection and self-doubt, Temple transformed her differences into strengths. Today she is well-known in the beef industry for improving some of the processes and equipment in slaughterhouses to make more humane experiences for cattle on their way to the industrial grinder.

Grandin's story reflects the archetype of the visionary, someone who sees beyond conventional boundaries and brings new possibilities to life. Her journey demonstrates the importance of self-mastery through self-acceptance, showing us that embracing our unique qualities--even those labeled as "weaknesses"--can lead to profound contributions to the world.

Taking Control of the Narrative: The Common Thread

Nick Vujicic, Jim Kwik, and Temple Grandin are all individuals who inspire me with their ability to transform their own lives and inspire others by transforming their unique challenges into opportunities. The common thread in their stories is the power of taking control of their narrative, choosing not to be defined by their circumstances but to redefine those circumstances into a source of strength and growth. They demonstrate that adversity is not something that we can avoid, so we can learn to embrace it and use it to make us uniquely strong. It is in those moments of struggle that we can rewrite our story and bloom into our full potential.

Part Three

Reflections & Anchors

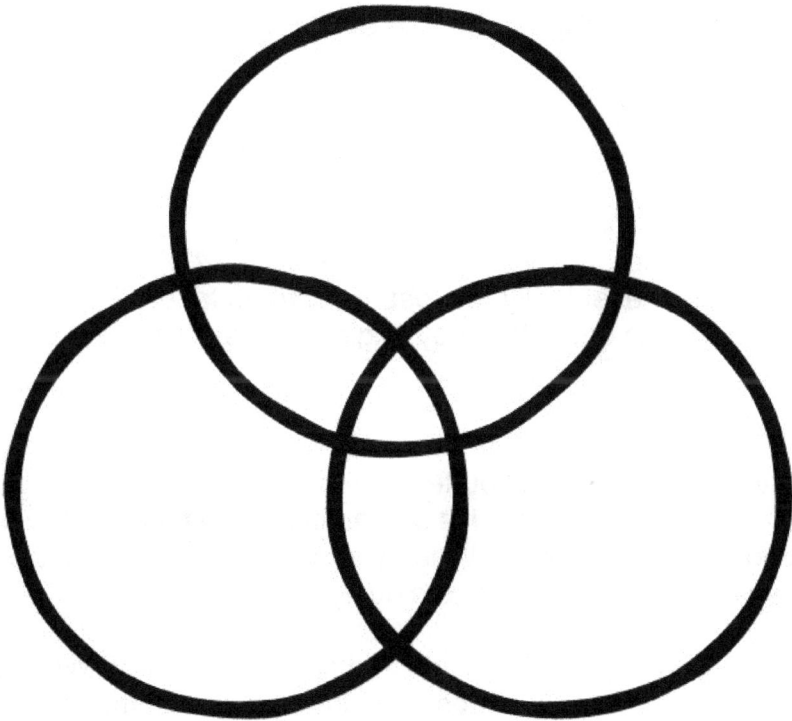

CHAPTER 7

THE WILD-WILD & YOUR BIG WHY

Mastering your future former self...

Did you ever do that project in school where you collected beautiful butterflies and maybe moths or beetles--pinning them to the back of a cardboard box? Maybe it was a class project, or perhaps you've seen one at the zoo? Even in a glass case, eventually, the beauty of them fades. The wings start to crumble. They begin to decay. They get dusty.

I often think of this when I think about the truth. To me, the truth is like a beautiful butterfly in many ways. It's delicate, and it needs to be free. It's a beautiful, living thing that lives among and through us. When we try to pin it down, it loses something. It eventually gets dusty.

The living truth needs to fly about and touch lots of flowers. Maybe sometimes it needs to migrate. Maybe sometimes it needs to hibernate. It needs to remain a bit wild, or it dies. We humans tend to want to pin it down, preserve it, know it. And yet, when we do that, something in it dies. It is no longer quite so perfect or wonderful. Eventually, it decays.

The Shift. Own your emotions; Own your life.

The truth is alive and evolving, and it needs to stay that way to remain the beautiful thing it is.

"Nothing well done is insignificant"

How we do one thing is, in some sense, how we do everything. Remember, it matters less where you start and much more that you start somewhere, sometime, somehow, and then pay attention to the results you get.

Once you start, you can measure your results against your expectations and desires and adjust accordingly. If you're lucky and put in the hard work, you will eventually begin to put the odds more and more in your favor.

…And then, and then…life, aging, things happen to kick you in the face. You find yourself thinking, "I might not make it," and you consider giving up. This is exactly when it's important to use the flip, use this as fuel to get to work.

Buck up, buttercup! Rally your internal courage and begin again.

"No plan survives first contact." Try not to take things personally. Life isn't designed to be easy most of the time, but you are designed to be resilient, adaptable, and able to learn and move forward.

Again, how successful you feel is more about the energetic state you approach things from than the specific things you do. Although what you do and who you do it with are also important factors to consider, how you bring yourself is most important. How well you get back up and dust yourself off when you get knocked down is the real key.

How you feel about yourself when you are by yourself is what really matters most. Try to remember, you are building a cathedral called 'the story of your life' and also 'the story of all life'.

The reset, the restart, gets more difficult as we age, and often the need for it becomes more acute, especially if you haven't practiced it. The flesh begins to get weak, though the spirit may still be willing. Nobody gets younger in this life. Nobody gets out alive.

Everything eventually decays and gets churned back into the stuff that creates new beginnings. So, start today. Live alive!

Begin where you are and do the best you can with what you have. Build on this, and over time you will find it gets easier and more natural with practice.

Cultivating Your Future Former Self

It's never too early (or too late) to start cultivating yourself into the person you want to be. One method I use is to focus on my future former self. This is slightly different from simply my future self.

My future former self is essentially me now, only in the context of who I will become. It is the self that looks back at myself and, hopefully, likes what I see. The self that now has a story that is upleveled, and told less defeatedly, while still being true, of course. If I follow the thought-loop all the way around, really my future former self is me, right now, yesterday, and tomorrow.

One way to cultivate your future former self is to imagine you are on your deathbed (should you be so lucky as to have a deathbed and the time and cognitive capacity to look back) and think about how you will view your life.

I find it more useful to think of myself in a year, five years, ten years, twenty years, and imagine looking back at myself today. What might I wish I had done differently? What might I wish I had spent more or less time doing? This helps me to step into who I want to be more immediately. Right now. Today.

What can you do today, that you will thank yourself for tomorrow?

Who and What Inspires You, and Why?

Another tool I like to use often is to pay attention to people who inspire me. Who inspires you? What is it about them that you admire? How can you cultivate more of those qualities in your own life?

It's not about being like someone else; it's about recognizing your values and using the reflection of others as clues about what you really value. Get more of that. Make more of that. Be more of that. Create more like that.

Of course, life has a vast array of challenges and potentials for you to step into, so it's not like you can expect to become a master and never struggle or face challenges again. It is reasonable to expect that you will get more comfortable with the challenges of life, however, and not let them knock you down so far when changes occur.

If you can make a habit of looking for the positive potential in everything that occurs, especially those that seem the most difficult to see as positive, you will be on a good path towards self-mastery.

One day you will still die. All the rest of the days, you will survive, and hopefully many of them, you will even vibrantly shine and thrive.

The Shift really is about making the best YOU out of the life you have. Maybe it's about dying in a state that does not add more trauma to the world and especially those around you. Maybe it's about approaching life more fully alive and experiencing it more vibrantly.

Remember that Self-Mastery is about cultivating a growth mindset (which means seeing failure as feedback, always looking for what life is teaching you), while also recognizing that there will be times when limiting beliefs and self-doubt will win out. It's about not wasting time and energy resisting the natural way things are, and instead, shifting readily without spending extra energy resisting.

Tune up the instrument that is your body and mind and routine regularly, and play. Engage with your life fully, wholeheartedly.

If you are feeling out of sorts, your body might be an un-played, underdeveloped instrument. When that happens, notice it and be glad you did. Then start playing!

Relax more and figure out what you need so you can give yourself more of that. In Western culture, often what we need is less 'stuff' and more open space, more unstructured time; more time to be wild.

When was the last time you danced, or sang unabashedly out loud?

The Shift. Own your emotions; Own your life.

Human history is full of remarkable examples of remarkable humans doing remarkable things. We consider them examples. In my lifetime and from my own culture, Keanu Reeves, Jim Carrey, Joe Rogan, Kevin Hart, Trevor Noah, Jacqualine Novogratz, Mary Morrison, Byron Katie, Zahra' Langhi, Malala Yousafzai, Dolly Parton, Dave Chappel, Chris White, Sean White... and many other speakers, comedians, innovators, artists, athletes, and philosophers come to mind. I think it is authentic expression and courage that I really admire most. For that reason, I also look up to many musicians. Chris Cornell, Beck, The Beatles, Prince, David Bowie-- so many legends in human history, even just from my lifetime.

The truth is, though, that the people who become famous or well-known for accomplishments are not the only or even the most remarkable humans in life. Human history is a weird phenomenon, and what gets held up into the light is not always the brightest or the first or the most of anything. In fact, what adds up to make something historical fact seems to have more to do with our collective shadows and traumas than things that are really worth celebrating most of the time.

It is actually our imperfections, our struggles, our 'flaws' which give our lives meaning and make those who succeed in the end most endearing to the rest of us.

When I think of who and what inspires me the most deeply, at the core of my being, it often has to do with courage and curiosity.

I think of my mentors over the years, like Mrs. Hazel, who grew prize-worthy dahlias and raised rabbits up the street from me when I was very young. She taught me a little about football, managing a grumpy husband, my period,

The Shift. Own your emotions; Own your life.

and 'familiar' pies (that's when there's not enough filling and the crusts are 'too close').

Beau, the beautiful dancer, musician, and teacher who was also my client for some years as I was her student. Just recently she made me get my dong quai powdered herb and put it into capsules and probably saved my life as I was deep in a 'hormonally enhanced' depression.

Kit, the gorgeous and graceful wise woman and former equine doula who enchanted me for a time with her strong convictions and her steel blue eyes. We spent many hours on her porch when she was hiring me to shop for her groceries after the lockdowns.

I think of Herb, the old man who lived two houses from me for a couple of decades and whom I used to clean for and helped through his wife's and his older brother's deaths and decline. He sang in a barbershop quartet and met other seniors at a coffee shop once a week to share jokes from the internet.

I think of my brother's son Benny, who died tragically before he turned 13 and inspired more people in his short life than many people you will meet. He was a great storyteller and a 'savage' liver of life.

I think of my friend Jaime, who was burned over 80% of his body in his teens, spent years in a military hospital getting skin graphs from the unburned parts onto the burned parts, and then ended up with a trust fund that purchased a house which many of us 'plaza rats', or street kids used as a safe place to go. He died in his late 30's from organ failure after just about 20 years of heavy drinking and not enough ability to sweat out toxins because of all the scaring…and the trust fund.

The Shift. Own your emotions; Own your life.

Jaime suffered a lot in some ways but in other ways he lived an incredible life. I never ever heard him say a disparaging word about anyone and I never heard him complain.

INVITATION TO ACTION: I invite you to reflect on these questions and write or record your reflections. Who do you look up to? What qualities and traits do they embody that you would like to bring more of into your life? What can you do today to be more like yourself?

There are far more remarkable examples that we will never hear of than there are famous ones. Even those whom we think of as 'famous' or infamous examples of what 'not' to do, or those who serve as warnings about how things can turn out if we do not tend to our own energy, have harnessed a type of mastery.

"Don't worry if you are not a success. At least you can serve as a bad example."

The things you become a master of are directly related to the things you regularly try and fail at. The difference is what energetic state you cultivate while you are failing and learning. Adopting the mindset that life is an infinite game and keeping yourself focused or returning your focus to what you want rather than what you don't want is an important key.

All of us are both examples and warnings, with the potential to be much more of both, depending on the choices we make and the beliefs we cultivate. How you perceive them

The Shift. Own your emotions; Own your life.

is always a clue about how you are perceiving yourself and your own life.

Pay attention, but not to criticize or put anyone else on a pedestal. Pay attention so you can better navigate your own life and alchemize the traumas that will otherwise pile up in your body and eventually stifle you.

It also matters how consciously we bring ourselves to our own lives. Get in touch with your underlying desires and unique talents, your special geniuses and gifts, so that you can develop them and bring them more fully into this world.

We need you to be you. No one else can. How much of you we get is up to you.

The Future of Humanity

We are all in this together. Ongoing throughout human history, and perhaps even before that, throughout the earth's history--or the history of life itself--we've faced what I call the "Chicken Little" conundrum: our ability to perceive and understand is minuscule in comparison to the vastness of the sky, and beyond.

Mass psychosis is a real problem these days and has been throughout human history. The degree and intensity of it rises and falls over time. Be aware that 'the masses' are often not very healthy or happy, and navigate this carefully and consciously.

I find that the best way to counter the mass psychosis that seems so prevalent in my lifetime is to be myself, authentically.

Spend time outside. Let yourself be a bit wild.

The Infinite Game

Domestication discourages you from thinking for yourself or developing your own unique perspective, but ultimately, 'the masses' need each of us to do our best to also be individuals. Yes, it can get tricky. Ideally, you can consider the masses and the future masses while also cultivating your own individuality.

I pose that even the fact that I've written and published this book, and that now you are reading it, is evidence that collectively and individually, you and I want to create a better and better future for our future offspring.

"The infinite game" is a concept that has been used for a long time to help put our dramas into a broader perspective. The ultimate mission is to keep the game going, not to win. When you begin to see it this way, you will start to create win-win-win situations all around you, and then the fun really begins!

Deviance and Wellness

Some degree of deviance is necessary for a healthy society. You might think of deviance as something negative, to be avoided, and it is true that too much of it can be fatal, but we need some of it to move forward. Life in totality evolves by holding a cohesive constant and also making slight deviations from the norm.

Your differences are your most valuable aspects. Do not let anyone else convince you that you must become more like everyone else. At the same time, it is true that learning to interact without creating tension and dysregulation is 'the name of the game.'

Being neurodivergent increases the odds of dysregulation in my own system and in the bodies of people around me. It took me until age 50 to realize this and begin to keep myself separate from other people in more conscious ways. The person who always pays for these interactions the most, at least from my perspective, is me. Rather than always trying to break down boundaries and barriers, I continue learning that they can be useful to protect others and allow me to best utilize my own energy.

Dogmatic Beliefs and The Wild-Wild

We cultivate ourselves in the images of gods and create gods in our own distorted images. Rising to god-like levels and filling the god-sized holes we've created for ourselves has become the preoccupation of civilization.

The Shift. Own your emotions; Own your life.

Nearly all governments, religions, and institutions will superimpose a framework over your being if you step into them, and this will naturally shrink your energetic state. They all eventually fall to the lowest common denominator. This is fine as a steppingstone, but institutions are notoriously limiting in their capacity to help you cultivate your highest potential, unless you recognize them as the rudimentary tools they are.

If you allow any institution to dictate your desires, tell you what is good and bad, right and wrong, and override your own capacity to decipher and choose, you will be reduced to this lowest common denominator state.

Dogmatic beliefs and practices can help bring stability and order into our lives, but they are also what has kept the masses in lower energetic states throughout most of human history.

If you want to bloom into your best and highest potentials, you will need to embrace what I call the "Wild-Wild" in yourself. This is a state of not knowing but trusting anyway. Ironically, religions often use this as a staple or guide, and then undermine the individual's capacity to trust or have faith in their own innate wisdom by dictating what or how or who they should trust or believe in. Rather than teaching us to cultivate this capacity in ourselves, many institutions teach us to hand over our trust and knowing for the dreary lull of conformity or "behaving".

It is crucial to consider what rules you follow blindly, and what standards you conform to. Recognize that you can choose to go against the grain, and that sometimes this will feel better, and sometimes it will feel worse. Only your own internal compass, your emotional guidance system, can tell you what is best for you in any given situation.

313

Mass Psychosis

The book, Stolen Focus: Why You Can't Pay Attention--and How to Think Deeply Again, by Johann Hari, does a great job of laying out the relationship between social media and the rise in ADHD. Since the publishing of that book in 2022 things only seem to be getting worse when it comes to our ability to focus or think straight.

It is obvious that this, along with the chemicals disrupting our endocrine and hormone systems, is causing rapid changes in our function, especially in our fertility and our sexuality. I imagine this will become an increasingly urgent issue in the coming years.

Where is the line between divergence or disorder and diversity? To me, it is a living line, like a flowing river, and to pretend it is a solid, unmovable, definitive thing seems silly. Of course, in navigating our individual lives, sometimes it is helpful to use a label that points to an inability or something we want help with. Like yin and yang, they exist in relativity, on a spectrum, and the extreme of one becomes the seed of the other.

Our institutions are very fond of using disempowering labels to identify those 'victims' who need help, the 'perpetrators' who are causing trouble, and then stepping in as the 'martyrs' who can fix things. Again, this is a very low energetic loop. If you want to live a truly fantastic life, you will need to pull yourself out of it more and more of the time.

I find that having a daily practice--at least once every day, but ideally two or three times every day--to spend time tending to my own energetic state, letting go of stresses and concerns that accumulate like lint in my pockets or between my toes, is an effective way to raise my vibrational and energetic state overall over time.

Just like personal hygiene practices and home maintenance are important to keep your physical body and external environment from becoming chaotic and unhealthy, if you make tending your energetic state a practice, you will find yourself in a much better place over time. Try it and find out!

Ceilings and Basements

Remember when we talked about your subconscious as an elephant and your consciousness as an ant? Consider that there are also high and low limitations that your subconscious has, which your consciousness can't see. If you try to become successful, but in your subconscious, you believe that money is the root of all evil or that rich people are greedy, for example, you will self-sabotage every time you get close to that ceiling.

If you believe that the only reason to ever take a day off is if you are ill or injured, and you don't give yourself any time to rest and recuperate, eventually you will find another way to get the time off you need by becoming ill or enduring an injury. If you believe that you are not worthy of love, you will get into relationships with people who are not capable of loving you and unconsciously reinforce this belief.

So, the way out of the basement is to raise your ceilings and also your floors. In general, it is helpful to expand your bandwidth of tolerance. This is tricky, as you don't want to train to tolerate lower and lower aspects of life, but at the same time, it's good to realize that life overall has floors much lower and ceilings much higher than yours can ever be. Expanding your bandwidth is a good way to think about it.

The Shift. Own your emotions; Own your life.

The floors are the lowest things we can tolerate. I was raised in poverty, for example, so my floors are much lower and dirtier than yours might be. I am also an American, so they are probably much higher than they might be if I lived in another country, so I am told.

Floors and ceilings don't only have to do with wealth and poverty, though. They have to do with relationships, and most importantly, our relationship with ourselves. It is more about what we tolerate from ourselves and others.

We all have our own unique sets of floors and ceilings, and most of them are beliefs we are not aware of, even though they are running our lives. How low and how high will we allow ourselves to go? This is an important bandwidth to pay attention to.

Remember, there is no one right or wrong way to be. If you are not happy with where or how you are, though, it is worth examining your floors and ceilings to see if they need expanding, contracting, or clarifying.

Beautiful Lies and Hard Truths

It's well known that we humans are prone to believing a beautiful lie over the hard truth. However, at some point, believing in beautiful lies creates even uglier truths, so in the long run, it is almost always best to get to the truth directly. Even if it stings a bit, it does, as they say, set you free.

With the truth, we can make decisions that are at least firmly rooted in the present moment. Remember to keep some open space around the truth at the same time, so it remains alive and does not become a dead, dusty butterfly.

The Shift. Own your emotions; Own your life.

Of course, plenty of mistakes will still be made, but when we are making mistakes with our footing firmly grounded in truth, those mistakes are much easier to navigate. When the relationships around us turn out to be fake, and the foundations of what we thought was true fall away to reveal that the people we were showing up for are not showing up for you, or that the people who taught you how to love didn't actually know how to do it very well themselves, then you are back at the start. It may be painful, but at least now your ant and your elephant are working together, and now, you can really get somewhere.

Here's a hard truth that might sting: If you are not happy with your life, then you and the rest of the people you are hanging out with are probably holding you back.

You will need to choose between holding on to the old and busted, yet familiar and sort of comfortable aspects of your life, and the great mysterious, fantastic, yet somewhat scary, completely unknown, and possibly out-of-your-control future.

There is likely going to be at least some periods of sitting alone with yourself, facing yourself, and uncomfortable discoveries of your own imperfections and self-deception.

"Routine and prejudice distort vision. Each man thinks his own horizon is the limit of the world." —Ancient Egyptian Proverb

Embracing Failure as Feedback

"I have not failed. I've just found 10,000 ways that won't work." — Thomas A. Edison

The Shift. Own your emotions; Own your life.

While it's important to have a goal or mission, make a plan, and prepare for your journey as best as you can, it's also important to recognize that you will fail. A lot. This does not mean it is futile to try. It does mean that it's important to 'enjoy the ride.' Spend the majority of your time doing things that satisfy you, even when you don't succeed. It is in the process of becoming who we want to be that the magic lies, not in having been.

The point is not to never make mistakes but to learn and improve along the way, and of course, to enjoy the journey itself. Failures are guaranteed; success is not. By learning to enjoy the process of learning, you will be building in an 'alternative' unavoidable type of success.

If your journey is epic, you will encounter many unexpected failures and successes, so your plan must be adjustable, malleable, and flexible. Get clear about your 'why' before you set out.

What values are you aiming to cultivate?

What is most important to you in this life?

What's the "big why" that motivates you?

In those times when all else becomes murky or incoherent, you can use this 'big why' as a guide to help you unfreeze, take action, and find more secure footing again.

Remember that acting is a key to moving through things more quickly. Keep in mind that stillness is also a valid option and sometimes helps us correct our alignment quickly too.

The Shift. Own your emotions; Own your life.

The truth is that your emotional dysregulation and overwhelming feelings are there to help guide you back on course.

Life has a funny way of constantly throwing curveballs at us, just when we think we've got it all figured out. That's why, to stay on track, we need something bigger than just short-term goals or ticking off items on a to-do list. We need to dig deeper and find our Big Why--the driving force that keeps us moving forward, even when the road gets bumpy. It's not about winning or losing; it's about playing the infinite game--a game with no final victory lap, just the continual unfolding of growth, purpose, and resilience.

Your Big Why

The concept of the Big Why is simple: it's your reason for getting out of bed each day, especially on those mornings when the snooze button feels like your best friend. Maybe it's the thing you live for. Maybe it's something you would die for. Psychologists call it intrinsic motivation, and research shows that having a clear sense of purpose or a "why" leads to greater resilience, perseverance, and well-being. A study published in The Journal of Positive Psychology found that individuals with a strong sense of purpose reported higher life satisfaction, greater emotional stability, and were more likely to overcome setbacks.

When my son and I participated in a local charter school called Family School, the students would choose a Big Why for each semester. All their major projects that semester would then be filtered through the lens of that Big Why. It made every project more engaging and enjoyable, which ultimately led to my son doing much more work but feeling like it was much easier.

Finding your Big Why is crucial because it gives meaning to the everyday grind and helps you connect your small, seemingly mundane actions to something much larger. It's like having your own personal GPS—when life's detours pop up (and they will), your Big Why recalculates the route, helping you stay on course.

The Living Truth: What's Real for You Right Now?

Life is messy, constantly changing, and full of contradictions. And that's where the living truth comes in. Unlike static truths, the living truth is dynamic--it evolves as you evolve. It's what's real for you right now, not necessarily what was true last year or even yesterday. The living truth demands that we stay flexible and curious, ready to adjust when new information or experiences come our way.

This flexibility is backed by cognitive-behavioral therapy (CBT), which emphasizes the importance of cognitive flexibility--the ability to shift our thinking and adapt to new perspectives. A study published in Behaviour Research and Therapy in 2016 found that people who cultivate cognitive flexibility are better equipped to manage stress, handle ambiguity, and navigate complex emotional landscapes. The living truth requires that we stay open to change, adapt to new realities, and recognize that our "truth" is always evolving.

Here's the kicker: the living truth often shows up when we're least expecting it, like in the middle of an argument when you suddenly realize, "Wait, maybe I'm the one who's wrong." Embracing this truth isn't about having all the answers; it's about being honest with ourselves, even when it's uncomfortable. After all, the more we face reality, the better equipped we are to move forward with clarity and intention.

The Shift. Own your emotions; Own your life.

Playing the Infinite Game: Making the Game Last

Now, let's talk about playing the infinite game. This idea, recently re-popularized by Simon Sinek, suggests that life isn't about reaching some final destination or "winning" once and for all. Instead, the infinite game is about staying in the game--continuing to grow, adapt, and evolve. In this game, the goal isn't to beat everyone else but to keep playing, learning, and expanding over time.

Research in positive psychology supports this concept, showing that people who focus on lifelong learning and growth report higher levels of well-being and satisfaction than those fixated on finite achievements like wealth or status.

A study published in Personality and Social Psychology Bulletin found that individuals who pursued growth-oriented goals--such as learning new skills or personal development--experienced more long-term happiness and emotional resilience compared to those focused solely on competitive or material goals.

In essence, playing the infinite game is about reframing our goals and expectations. It's realizing that there's no "final level" in life, no ultimate finish line. The real win comes from embracing the ongoing process of growth, from learning to enjoy the journey rather than just fixating on the destination. When we play the infinite game, we stop chasing perfection and start focusing on progress. We learn to love the grind, not just the reward.

The Shift. Own your emotions; Own your life.

Our the Big Why's keep us grounded in purpose, the living truth keeps us adaptable and honest with ourselves, and playing the infinite game ensures that we never stop learning, growing, and evolving. After all, life isn't a sprint-- it's a marathon that we run in waves, sometimes soaring on highs, sometimes weathering lows, but always moving forward, one step at a time.

Summary of Chapter Seven

Keep Your Eyes on the Prize.

Ultimately, how we live is reflected in the stories we repeat. So, get out there and live fully. Do your best to be wise.

Use the right tool for the right job, and if something isn't working, stop and make a change.

Recognize that you are both dumber and smarter than you think.

You can learn new things and make changes—in fact, you are always changing. How consciously and deliberately you do so is up to you.

"Before enlightenment: Chop wood, carry water. After enlightenment: Chop wood, carry water."

Regardless of how much we agree or disagree on various points, the fact remains: there is always much work to be done in this life. The great thing about that is through work, we can solve most of our personal and societal problems, and if we're lucky, survive long enough to create new ones.

When choosing your enemy wisely (as in, with the aim of 'what works'), may I suggest that you consider making your own mediocrity or smallness the enemy? Not in the sense of being an enemy you wish to destroy, but rather as an adversary you want to outshine, outrun, outlive. To this end, dear brave heart, I trust we will find each other in good company.

It's important to celebrate your small and big wins all along the way. Get into the habit of noticing when you get things right to counter the waves and voices that will try to sway you back into believing you can't, you shouldn't, no one ever has, or whatever limiting belief your 'council of apes'-- or pre-programmed limited beliefs--is throwing at you. Keep a journal, a folder, or a scrapbook of evidence of wins--nice things people say or do for you, nice things you do or say for others, the times you get a long run of green traffic lights, that incredible smile a baby gives you from the shopping cart at the grocery store, finding a perfectly shaped apple.

There are no wrong answers, and nothing is too big or too small. The point is to train your nervous system to notice things that feel good, things that affirm you are safe and loved and living in an abundant, joyful universe.

The truth is a fluid, living thing that exists in the present moment. The stories we tell about what happened to us or what we think is going to happen are all projections and not the real thing.

Remember that life is that special, magic, ever-fleeting thing that happens in the space between things--in the present moment, in the choices we make now, and now, and now.

You cannot pre-plan it all out, and what if you could? You cannot capture it, pin it down, and define it for all time. It has to breathe, it has to fly, it has to grow and change, and be allowed to dance in order to be alive. Just like you.

The Shift. Own your emotions; Own your life.

Real People Who Inspire Many:

Wangari Maathai: The Environmental Visionary

Wangari Maathai was a Kenyan environmentalist, feminist, and the first African woman to win the Nobel Peace Prize. Her story is one of resilience, vision, and the transformative power of grassroots action.

Born in 1940 in rural Kenya, Wangari grew up in a community deeply connected to the land. However, as colonial agricultural practices took root, deforestation and environmental degradation began eroding traditional ways of life. This shaped her early awareness of the importance of environmental conservation.

Wangari pursued her education with relentless determination, earning a doctorate--the first woman in East or Central Africa to do so--and becoming a professor. However, her journey wasn't easy. She faced cultural opposition, sexism, and political resistance throughout her life.

In 1977, Wangari founded the Green Belt Movement, a grassroots initiative to combat deforestation by planting trees. Initially, her goal was practical: to restore degraded land, provide firewood, and improve agricultural productivity for women in rural communities. Over time, the movement grew into a symbol of resistance against environmental destruction, inequality, and corrupt governance.

Through the Green Belt Movement, Wangari empowered Kenyan women, teaching them to plant trees and take ownership of their communities' natural resources. Despite facing imprisonment, harassment, and political opposition,

326

she persisted, planting over 50 million trees and inspiring environmental movements globally.

Wangari embodies the archetypes of the Visionary and the Warrior. Her ability to see the interconnectedness of environmental, social, and economic issues was revolutionary, while her willingness to confront systemic corruption demonstrated immense courage. She faced the shadow of fear head on--fear of authority, failure, and personal harm. By confronting these fears, she integrated her shadow and transformed it into unshakable resolve.

Wangari's legacy is one of hope and empowerment. She reframed deforestation and environmental degradation as solvable problems, showing that collective action could create lasting systemic change.

Zahra' Langhi: A Modern Bridge Builder

Zahra' Langhi is a Libyan peace activist, feminist, and co-founder of the Libyan Women's Platform for Peace (LWPP). Her work is deeply rooted in integrating spiritual and cultural wisdom into modern peace-building efforts, embodying the themes of reconciliation, shadow integration, and collective healing.

Born and raised in Libya, Zahra' Langhi grew up witnessing the struggles of her country, including authoritarianism, conflict, and the marginalization of women. Her education and spiritual upbringing inspired her to seek a better way, blending traditional values with modern activism. During Libya's 2011 revolution, she became an advocate for women's inclusion in the country's rebuilding process, recognizing that sustainable peace required diverse voices.

In 2011, Langhi co-founded the LWPP, an organization dedicated to advancing women's leadership in Libya's political and social spheres. She drew on archetypes of feminine wisdom--collaboration, empathy, and inclusivity--arguing that peace could not be achieved through violence or exclusion. Her platform emphasized dialogue, education, and nonviolence as pathways to healing.

Langhi also introduced the concept of "Masculine and Feminine Paradigms of Leadership," advocating for a balance of assertive and nurturing qualities in political decision-making. Her work sought to counteract the shadow of patriarchal dominance and militarization, proposing a holistic approach to reconciliation.

Malala Yousafzai: Education as a Living Truth

Malala Yousafzai's story also embodies what it means to live in alignment with a *Big Why*. Her courage didn't spring from a desire for fame or recognition--it came from her unshakable belief that education is a right, not a privilege. As a young girl living under the oppressive rule of the Taliban, Malala was determined to go to school, knowing deep inside that her education wasn't just about her--it was about creating a ripple effect for other girls, for future generations. She felt the injustice of being denied something so fundamental and decided that her truth--her *Big Why*--was worth risking everything for.

The Shift. Own your emotions; Own your life.

In The Shift, we talk about how living your truth is about taking responsibility for your life, owning your choices, and not waiting for someone else to grant you permission to live out your purpose. Malala didn't wait for the world to change; she became the catalyst for that change. Even when a Taliban gunman tried to silence her, she emerged even stronger, speaking not just for herself but for every child denied the chance to learn.

Mo Gawdat: Happiness Through Awareness and Growth

A former Chief Business Officer at Google X, Mo Gawdat is a tech visionary who faced an unimaginable personal loss when his son, Ali, passed away suddenly at the age of 21. This tragedy propelled him into a journey of self-discovery and healing, culminating in his groundbreaking book, *Solve for Happy*.

Mo's philosophy of happiness revolves around understanding how the mind works, managing expectations, and aligning with a higher purpose. He teaches that emotional resilience is not about avoiding pain but learning to process and grow from it. His message is rooted in both science and spirituality, blending rationality with deep emotional insight. Mo exemplifies the archetype of the Sage, sharing his hard-earned wisdom to help others navigate life's challenges with grace and intention.

Mo's journey explores the deeper meaning behind our actions and the pursuit of long-term fulfillment. His teachings emphasize that happiness and growth are

The Shift. Own your emotions; Own your life.

ongoing processes that require reflection, emotional regulation, and a willingness to face life's shadows. Mo's life is a reminder that even the greatest tragedies can become catalysts for wisdom, purpose, and connection.

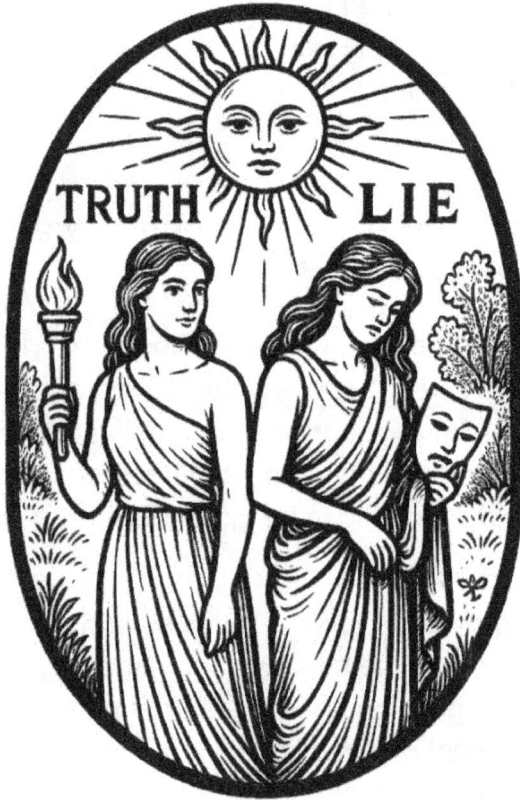

The Naked Truth and the Beautiful Lie

This is an age-old tale in which Truth and Lie crossed paths near a stream. Lie, sly and full of charm, suggested they go for a swim, promising cool waters and a refreshing escape. Truth, ever trusting, agreed and undressed, leaving her clothes on the bank. But as Truth swam, Lie seized the moment, slipping into Truth's garments and walking into the world, disguised as the very thing she was not.

When Truth emerged, she found her clothes gone and Lie parading through the streets, convincing everyone she was the real thing. Truth, exposed and vulnerable, had a choice: cover herself with Lie's falsehoods or remain naked, stripped of all but her authenticity. She chose to remain bare, standing in her discomfort because she knew that dressing herself in lies would only mask the reality of who she was.

As Lie walked through life, many welcomed her, preferring the dressed-up version of reality to the rawness of truth. People were drawn to Lie's comfort and ease, avoiding the unsettling confrontation that the naked Truth brought with her.

But Truth, in her nakedness, was still alive. Though she was difficult to face and even harder to accept, she was the living essence of reality, where transformation begins. Lie, for all her charm, was like a dead butterfly pinned to the back of a cardboard box--beautiful in form but hollow and devoid of the vitality that Truth carried. In time, those seeking real growth found themselves drawn to Truth, recognizing that only she could bring the kind of change that mattered.

331

The Shift. Own your emotions; Own your life.

332

The Shift. Own your emotions; Own your life.

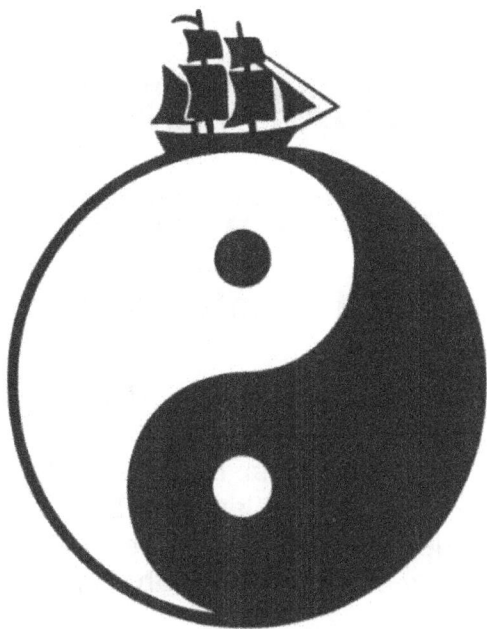

CHAPTER 8

"GET SUM ON YA!"

Putting it all into practice…

Take action and iterate!

Here we are, at the end again. Keep in mind, every ending carries the potential for countless new beginnings. I hope this conclusion leaves you with a sweet finish and a lingering afterglow of personal growth and empowerment.

We have crossed a mighty river together in the pages of this book. It's natural that you might feel a bit soaked. Take heart. All of this will soften and solidify over time. I hope you revisit the tools we've discussed and continue to polish and cultivate your unique toolkit as you develop a more vibrant life.

As you live more in alignment with your values, and as the ant of your consciousness becomes more coherently aligned with the elephant of your subconscious and superconscious, you will navigate the turbulence between your desires and the constant murmurs of the 'overculture', or the "underculture" as the case may be.

The Shift. Own your emotions; Own your life.

You are learning to discern when to push forward with wisdom and when to take great leaps. You are learning to lean into the upswings when you feel fired up and to act more cautiously when you notice the impulse to slow down.

You are beginning to understand that you can use your own thoughts, feelings, breath, and other tools to deliberately and consciously shift your energy, tune yourself to higher levels of existence, and bring yourself into greater alignment.

By now, you are likely realizing more and more often that your life is entirely your responsibility. You are catching more frequent glimpses of how your circumstances and story are, at least in large part, of your own making.

Of course, there are circumstances in life you can't control, but you can control how you respond to them. How you engage with life is up to you. Perhaps you've recognized some areas where you've been holding yourself back and have begun asking yourself those important questions:

What do I really want?

What is really true?

What would be best for me to DO, right now?

Is this moving me closer or further from my goals and becoming the type of person I want to be?

You have discovered that The Shift is yours to cultivate, practice, and master. Remember, mastery is an ongoing process, not a destination. Now it is up to you to take this knowledge and apply it to your life in ways that only you can determine.

The Shift. Own your emotions; Own your life.

I trust that you will use this knowledge wisely.

"Play It Again!"

The Shift is not a one-time event. It's not a destination. It's something you can practice and improve. The best examples of humanity are those who have learned to make the shift often and well, navigating the twists and turns of life with authentic style, grace, and ease.

We exist on a continuum between the infinitesimal and the astronomical. Our lives pass by much faster and slower than you might think at any given time. Your frame-rate will change throughout your lifetime. What seems impossible can become inevitable, and often things that seem like certain bets turn out to be mere flashes in the night.

Sanity and satisfaction are all about the relationships you have with yourself and with humanity at large. In some ways, it never ends, and you can't get it wrong. In other ways, everything is finite, and everything you do matters.

When you stay open to possibilities, the truth is alive and always evolving through you. You are part of an ever-evolving process of life iterating itself. It's up to you to make the most of it.

With mainstream society often acting incoherently, steeped in lies and illusions, and living in a perpetual state of dysregulation, disempowerment, and disease, it's tricky to keep your body coherent and regulated, and it might be more important than ever.

As the rapid adoption of large language models (LLMs) and other "AI"s (artificial intelligences) changes our lives at such

The Shift. Own your emotions; Own your life.

a pace that our grandchildren are likely to live in a world
that is currently inconceivable to us now, it seems crucial
that we don't lose sight of this basic aspect of being
human.

When dealing with 'humanity at large,' recognize that most
humans are not fully conscious most of the time. The
majority are acting from rudimentary default programming,
focusing on the negative, which unfortunately creates a lot
of misery.

Remember that belonging and fitting in are not the same.
You belong to life. You are part of humankind, which is part
of nature. All this is evolving, and we are on the leading
edge of creation.

You only owe yourself your most authentic self. The goal is
not to 'fit in', but to remember who you really are, take up
all the space you need, and bloom into your best self
completely. When you make your own regulation and
coherence a priority, navigating life will become easier over
time.

"Large questions get us a larger life." —James Hollis

We've covered a lot together on this journey. By now,
you've realized that the biggest problem in your life is most
often you. Hopefully you see that much of your own
suffering stems from a lack of emotional fitness and
personal responsibility for your energetic and emotional
states. Hopefully you also see that you can improve your
life and reduce your own suffering by becoming more
emotionally fit.

Remember, you are not alone in this. It's a natural part of
the human condition. Your tendency to self-sabotage and
make things harder than they have to be are patterns that

The Shift. Own your emotions; Own your life.

most humans have shared throughout human history. We are all in this together; and we all can improve. Many, though not all, of the details of your life are up to you.

We reviewed how taking responsibility is the most powerful and courageous step you can take when your life isn't where you want it to be.

Hopefully, you've decided how to design your future self and spent time envisioning your potential future life.

Take a good, honest look at yourself. Then be determined and resolve to work to set yourself free. Do your best and allow yourself to be humble and human.

The good news about realizing that your energetic state colors everything in your life—and that your energetic state is your responsibility—is that you can reclaim much of your power over the details of your life. You can play a more conscious role in your perceptions of those details. **Remember, with great responsibility comes great power!**

"Life is a short pause between two great mysteries." —Carl Jung

I hope you joined me in building your personalized emotional fitness toolkit and made a public declaration for additional accountability. You have everything you need to start improving your emotional fitness today and continue for the rest of your life. I trust I've convinced you that it's worth it, that you are worth it, and that you can do it. I probably didn't need to convince you that the alternative is worse.

I hope you've started tracking your progress and are noticing your self-defeating patterns and habits by now,

338

The Shift. Own your emotions; Own your life.

and that you continue to adjust and refine your habits as you learn what works best for you. Remember, this is an ongoing process, not a single destination.

Be patient with yourself, especially when it feels like you're spinning your wheels. If that happens, just take a deep breath, exhale, and begin again. Reach out for support when you need it.

Consider becoming a mentor or supporting figure in someone else's life. Helping and teaching others is an excellent way to expand and hone your own skills.

Keep in mind that emotional resilience is built in The Shift--in the gap between realizing you're off course or dysregulated and bringing yourself back to coherence. Step back, pause, and reframe your story as often as you need to. Let go of the stories that no longer serve you as you build a better life.

Laugh more. Love more. Play more. Lighten up a little more.

Consider the alternatives, but not too long.

Check in with yourself often to ensure you're being kind and not overly harsh or judgmental. Criticism and cynicism won't help you become the best version of yourself.

Remember to use both small, steady, incremental steps and giant leaps. Vary it up!

Use what works for you and always take time to pause and question.

Don't be afraid of your shadow; know it is always with you, and it serves a purpose like all things do.

The Shift. Own your emotions; Own your life.

When things feel stagnant or hopeless, shift your perspective, clean your room, visit a friend, or take a walk outside.

Observe the other people and creatures in life to regain a healthy perspective.

Pause, breathe, and reset. Hum. Shake. Drink some cool water or warm tea. Raise your vibration internally, and things will look and feel different. Prioritize your energetic state and mind the gaps between where you think you are and where you want to be as invitations to grow into new and improved versions of yourself.

Remember, you are not what happened to you. You are what is wanting to express itself through you.

This is how we become our full, truest, most authentic, and highest potential selves.

"The spirit of evil is the negation of the life force by fear. Only BOLDNESS can deliver us from evil. If the risk is not taken, the meaning of life is violated." —Carl Jung

First, we ride. Then we die.

In between so many 'micro deaths,' we become what we are, what we can be, and sometimes what we never imagined we could be. This is living a fantastic, inspired, creative life. This is how we can ensure our existence contributes to the light.

The SHIFT Method & SHIFT Lab

The work that came before this book and went into publishing this book led to the creation of a simple SHIFT Method that anyone can apply to get better results from their life. The SHIFT method is a framework based on these lessons. It can be applied to individual and group settings and involves Seeing your Story, Hold a safe space or hearing what it you are really saying, Investigating and inviting the feeling in, Feeling the feeling without giving it power, and Transforming the vulnerability and confusion into clarity and strength.

The SHIFT Lab has naturally arisen from that, as a place we can collaborate and share what works best and where we get stuck along the way. Please join us or any other group of humans for support and encouragement when you are ready.

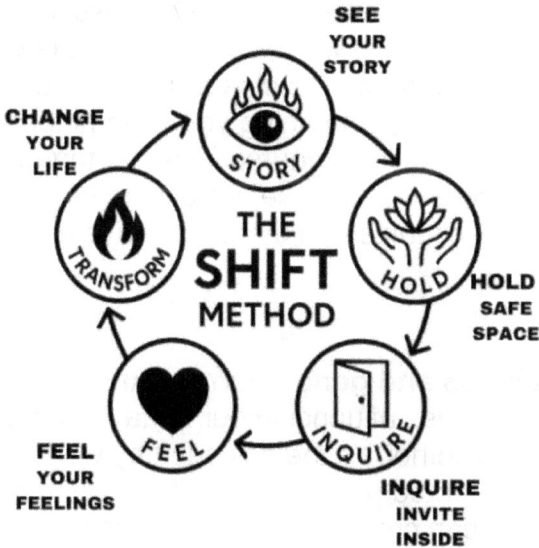

SEE YOUR STORY

CHANGE YOUR LIFE

THE SHIFT METHOD

HOLD SAFE SPACE

FEEL YOUR FEELINGS

INQUIRE INVITE INSIDE

341

The Obstacles You Have Overcome

The most significant obstacle we all face is our own limiting beliefs. Our default mode often involves getting in our own way and making things harder than they need to be. Self-doubt and the belief that we are not worthy or capable of making the changes we desire are the first and last hurdles to overcome.

In a society that sometimes seems bent on celebrating disease and dysfunction, maintaining coherence and alignment with wellness and wholeness can be challenging. We are all in this together. The work you are doing matters. Thank you for taking the time to develop your own strategies and toolkit for greater emotional fitness and satisfaction with your life.

Not only does your past not have to hold you back, but it can become fuel to help you reach higher levels of conscious evolution in this life. Find the lessons and examples that resonate with you and always remember that when you see someone else's shadow, you are probably also seeing something you have hidden from, shamed, or denied within yourself. Rather than criticize others, appreciate that we see our own reflections in one another, and recognize that there is always much work to be done.

Hidden traumas and generational abuses subtly permeate our lives, influencing our behaviors and interactions. Whether it's the scars left by war, internal conflicts, or inherited patterns of dysfunction, these deep-seated issues can create significant challenges.

Acknowledging and addressing these hidden wounds is crucial for genuine healing and growth. Every generation

342

seems to have their own, and ours are underway and on schedule. Understanding their impact allows us to break free from destructive cycles and fosters a healthier, more coherent existence.

Conflict Resolution and Change Management

Life is inherently filled with conflicts and the need for change management and resolutions. Navigating these effectively requires emotional intelligence, patience, and adaptation.

Developing these skills can transform how we handle disputes, adapt to new circumstances, and manage personal growth. Embracing conflict resolution as a storytelling process can also help us make sense of our experiences and integrate them into our personal narratives in more meaningful ways.

Life can be difficult, especially for those of us who come from a culture of poverty mindset or victim mentality. Give yourself and those around you plenty of grace and compassion. Shifting your level of consciousness is a process that takes time.

Recognize that you may have spent much time practicing 'improper techniques,' so resetting your default energetic state from negative and forceful to neutral and receptive could take extra time.

Eventually, you will begin to cultivate more positivity and tap into your inherent personal power with greater ease and speed. This doesn't mean you won't face challenging situations or experience frustration or dysregulation ever again. It does mean you can learn to respond in ways that prevent those lower energetic states from routinely ruling or ruining your life.

The Techniques You Have Learned

I've introduced simple tools techniques that have been most helpful in my own journey of self-mastery and emotional fitness. Pause, Question, Breathe & Release. Consume less. Move and feel more. These are always available to all of us, although they take practice to have them come naturally.

Sound Healing, Dance, Temperature Change, Hot and Cold Showers, Perspective Reframes, Letting Go of Expectations, Laughter, Movement, Shaking, Rhythm, Harmony, Realigning with Purpose, Clearing Clutter, Journaling, Meditation, Documenting, Doodling, Contemplation, Compassionate Touch, Neurographic Art, Qi Gong, Yoga, Appreciation, Gratitude, and Helping Others are all effective tools that any of us can use almost anytime, for free. I hope you will try some of them and find at least a few that are helpful for you.

They don't need to be done in any particular order, and you don't need to do all of them.

Often just one tool is enough to shift you into a better state where you can move forward with better outcomes.

Also remember, these are not the only tools available to you. There are many additional tools and techniques I encourage you to explore. Find what works for you and let go of whatever does not serve you in your present journey forward.

The Shift. Own your emotions; Own your life.

Now that you understand that The Shift is not a one-time act or a destination, you can choose to make it a way of being. The Shift is a decision to be present in the NOW and to use perspective to navigate life more calmly and coherently.

You will still have ups and downs, but the degree, length, and intensity of suffering you endure can be significantly decreased. You can make better plans for your life and relationships and see the fruition of your efforts, rather than spinning your wheels and repeatedly getting the same messy results.

Get clear on your personal values and regularly check the alignment of your 'elephant' (subconscious) and your 'ant' (conscious). See if you can also harmonize and play well with others in the fields of your broader environment and the context of your place in history and society (superconscious).

Allow yourself to become more coherent by giving yourself grace when you realize you are out of coherence. Remember that 'what we resist, persists', so rather than trying not to become dysregulated, just learn to recognize when you are and gently bring yourself back to a more regulated state. Aim for progress, not perfection.

Regularly checking your daily actions and habits against your underlying values and updating them as necessary, will naturally build a satisfying and fulfilling life, regardless of the details, obstacles, and struggles you encounter.

The victim-perpetrator-martyr mentality is a natural default, at least in our current culture, so don't beat yourself up or feel ashamed when you fall back into it. Shame and blame will only keep you stuck. Instead, congratulate yourself when you recognize you are slipping and use it as fuel to rise from your own ashes once again.

Look to people you admire for inspiration, but do not place them on a pedestal. Recognize that anything you see in someone else reflects something within you. This applies to both those you criticize or judge and to those you admire. Look for those qualities in yourself, learn to forgive yourself and others for perceived imperfections, and always work to become the most functional and coherent human you can be.

Try to remember you are having a biological, physical experience; and also, a metaphysical, energetic experience. Your emotions and resulting feelings are valuable information that can help you navigate the complex oceans of reality when you learn to interpret and process them more effectively.

There is much more going on than you are consciously aware of or capable of fully comprehending. Some of the data you get is naturally going to be misinterpreted. It's important to hold your own opinions loosely and be curious about other perspectives.

There are many languages you do not understand. Learn to recognize that your emotions, feelings, and intuitions are not facts, but they are a language that your body speaks, and they can be clues and messages to help guide you towards a more fulfilling and satisfying life.

Learn to incorporate all information into your understanding and let go of whatever does not serve you in your current journey. Let go of what is not serving you. Cultivate what brings you fulfillment and coherence.

The Shift. Own your emotions; Own your life.

Trust that the right things and people and ideas will come into your awareness at the right time, and practice becoming as physically and emotionally fit as you can be.

People & Perspectives

The personal stories I've shared from a first-person perspective are true to the best of my knowledge and recollection. I've tried to minimize personal details about others because they are not here to share their side of the story, and I have done my best to be compassionate to all perspectives.

I hope that the person you've met most on this journey is yourself. While it's crucial to find role models and get clear about the qualities you do and don't want to emulate, ultimately, this journey is about becoming your fullest, most alive, and authentic self.

I highly recommend diving deeper into the life stories of those I've mentioned or anyone else who inspires you. I encourage you to think about your own life story, and how you would like it to be. No human on earth has escaped the struggles with identity and self-sabotage we all face.

Keep a mental note of what inspires you and store these as tools you can draw on whenever needed. More importantly, keep a record of your own successes--times when you triumphed over difficult circumstances. Reflect on them whenever you need a reminder of your resilience and ability to navigate challenges.

Your popularity and approval will ebb and flow. In fact, when you go against the grain, you may encounter significant friction. Exceptional success often requires

The Shift. Own your emotions; Own your life.

being disliked and criticized. Remember, true consciousness does not follow the herd. It requires comfort with discomfort and an appreciation for being unappreciated at times.

Exercises & Practice

The tools you've practiced--Breathing, Pausing, Questioning, Shifting your breath, Shifting Perspective, Reflecting on Mindset (mind your mind), Letting Go of Limiting Beliefs, Setting Aligned Goals, Building Good Systems of Support, and Moving your body--are foundational. These are foundational strategies, as are deciding to take personal responsibility, taking radical personal responsibility for your own actions and inactions, documenting and tracking your progress, and adjusting as you build resilience. I hope you will always keep these in your toolkit.

Remember, action is usually better than standing still, but recognize that charging forward in the wrong direction can lead you astray. Regularly check in with yourself and correct your course when you feel off.

When in doubt, take your foot off the gas, listen to your heart, and recalibrate. Practice breathing and cleaning up after yourself, both literally and figuratively. Sometimes, doing the mundane, like washing the dishes, can help you find clarity when you're unsure of your next move.

The tools presented in this book are a gallery of options for you to choose from, think about, and modify to fit your unique path. There is no single correct way to navigate life. Your journey will require you to adapt and sometimes create your own methods.

The Shift. Own your emotions; Own your life.

If something isn't working, don't waste energy pushing against it. **Remember, failure isn't your enemy-- stagnation is.** Fear and a fixed mindset are the real challenges, but they are also invitations to grow.

Holding two seemingly conflicting ideas in mind at the same time is essential to effectively navigate life's waves. Our perceptions are limited, and our brains are wired to default towards fear and suspicion.

Make sure that whatever else happens, at the very least, you are always on your side.

Asking good questions is key to success. Regularly ask yourself:

Is this really true?

Why do I think or feel this?

What is the deeper truth here?

What is perfect about this?

How does this serve me?

What is trying to come through me?

What do I really, really want?

Radical Responsibility & A Growth Mindset; Cultivating Your Custom Toolkit

We've covered a lot of tools and information in this book, and my hope is that you take away just one or two things that resonate with you right now. Don't be distracted by what doesn't feel relevant or useful in the moment.

Trust that this information is now within you, and it will surface when you're ready to use it--at the right time, in the right way.

Taking personal responsibility for your own life and deciding to actively shift your mindset and ultimately shift your life story is a radical act of self-love. Ultimately, I believe it is the most valuable gift you can give yourself and all the rest of humanity. No one else can bring the unique combination of gifts and style that is simmering inside you.

I hope this book is a helpful guide or at least provides some sparks to ignite your own healing journey and build your own custom tool kit for mastering your emotions so that you can be more of a master in every aspect of your life.

The tools and techniques themselves are less important than the mindset and energy you bring to them. That's why this book is called *The Shift*.

Your ability to recognize when you're feeling out of alignment and to use the appropriate tool to bring yourself back to a functional state will improve with practice. This is a foundational skill that can make every other aspect of your life better.

Over time using the best tools for you will become more natural, just like daily habits like brushing your teeth or

The Shift. Own your emotions; Own your life.

tying your shoes has become--some of them will start to become automatic.

Please don't give up if you become frustrated or start to feel hopeless if it is difficult or even feels impossible sometimes, especially at first. This is natural. It's part of the process. It happens to everyone, and it too shall pass. It will get easier with practice.

There are others ready and willing to help you, but saving you is not up to them. Only you can save yourself. When you need to, take a step back--think of it as a little "cha-cha-cha"--and keep moving forward.

Dare to dance!

Heart to Heart of the Purple Onion

Like layers of a beautiful, sweet, purple onion, my own evolution has come in waves and old versions of myself have peeled off and left behind like dry, discarded snake skins.

There have been times in my life when I have felt lost, fragmented, separated, hopeless, damaged, ruined, broken, unloved, unworthy of love…and other times in my life when I have managed to take great leaps, or steady small steps, and felt triumphant in my accomplishments.

I have felt powerful and weak. I have broken my bones with my own force, and I have coaxed mountains with the power of playful dancing through fresh snow.

I have earned degrees, transformed properties, produced original songs, published books, raised a healthy and kind son, and much, much more.

I have also struggled with severe mental and physical health challenges, ruined relationships, and felt the sting that comes with knowing I did not bring my best self to the situation at hand more than once.

I have also worked with hundreds of clients and students who have struggled with similar challenges and opportunities to grow, heal, and bloom into new iterations of themselves.

I deeply desire for you to become fully the unique being that only you can be. I believe we can live far more vibrantly and fantastically than we often see in humanity today.

The Shift. Own your emotions; Own your life.

Your unrealized potential lies waiting to bloom from the very shadows where you currently struggle. I invite you to examine your patterns, your recurring failures or complaints, and find that Shift within yourself.

Open more space in yourself and in your story. Make room for new possibilities. Loosen your grasp on what you're sure is true, and consider that there is much more within you yet to be discovered. Remember it is easy for us to be deceived and even easier for us to deceive ourselves. Also remember to give yourself some grace, practice humility and patience, and embrace the journey of the process.

We humans can easily become trapped in our limited perceptions. We can start believing there is no magic or mystery beyond what we can see.

When we turn back in fear or doubt, we forfeit those golden opportunities. We miss out on sharing those gifts that only we can bring to humanity. It is up to each of us to discover and cultivate the unique ways that we can best contribute to the collective.

Remember there is always more potential than we can fully step into in any given moment. This potential creates the very tension necessary to propel all of existence forward. There is no point in regret or lamenting opportunities missed, and there is also no shame in giving a heartfelt apology anytime one is due.

The present moment is all there ever is, and it is the sum of so many butterfly smiles and hummingbird whispers. It could not be any other way.

Those moments in life that are the most meaningful, the most delicious, and the richest are the moments that our emotions, if we choose to listen to them, can guide us

The Shift. Own your emotions; Own your life.

toward. The deepest, most fulfilling, and most meaningful and rewarding aspects of life often lie on the other side of doing hard things. One of the hardest, yet most rewarding, is learning to face and navigate our emotional states in a nuanced way, rather than dismissing intense emotions as 'too much' or disruptive.

We are nearly at the end of this part of our journey together, dear and brave one, but the broader journey of navigating this life is nowhere near its end.

Remember, you are more than the sum of your parts, and there are aspects of yourself you've yet to discover. I know this is true because in my life I have experienced many iterations of transformation and self-realization.

We Are All in This Together.

In today's world, the boundaries between issues seem increasingly blurred and easy to stumble over. Many people feel so overwhelmed that they resort to coping strategies that involve checking out of reality, distracting themselves with mindless entertainment, or immersing themselves in addictive behaviors. It's as if we've forgotten how to communicate on a deeper level, beyond the polarizing topics of politics, religion, gender, insurance, disorders, and healthcare.

Currently, conversations that venture beyond the superficial often become battlegrounds, steeped in personal insults and vitriol. Once-taboo topics have now become the primary subjects of discussion, with extremes becoming the norm. It feels as though we are constantly swinging between opposites, unable to find balance so much of the time.

The Shift. Own your emotions; Own your life.

Addiction has expanded far beyond substances like alcohol, weed, fentanyl, and ketamine. We are also addicted to disempowering mindsets, television programming, social media, sugar, caffeine, and even the drama that comes with a cycle of blame and shame. Negative thinking and limiting beliefs, rooted in victim, savior, martyr, or perpetrator mentalities like the broken father and the death mother archetypes, fuel this cycle.

Nearly everyone has someone or something to blame for why they can't fully be who they want to be, often because they feel compelled to help someone else who needs them. Chronic illness, disabilities, and a string of diagnosed dysfunctions have become increasingly common and even popular. It all feels truly sick and sickening.

The truth is that much of this is self-perpetuating and self-created. This is actually 'good news', because it means we can create positive changes by deciding to take different actions in our individual lives.

I believe this Shift begins with learning to recognize dysregulation and developing a healthier relationship with our own emotions and energetic bodies.

It is easier than you might think to make this much needed internal shift. We can do it individually and collectively. We can find steady, calm, coherent, friendly footing again. **It starts with a very small, very significant shift.**

We are capable of so much more than just being "okay." We have the potential to be fantastic, to rise to greatness. We have the potential to become superhuman, or at least, to create better lives for ourselves, and better systems for future humans.

The Shift. Own your emotions; Own your life.

To survive and thrive through the shifts and technological advances on the horizon, we need to elevate our ability to manage stress and learn to cope in healthier ways. A healthy mind and body can let go of things and move past them. With practice, we can learn to alchemize our emotions, process them, and compartmentalize them in healthy ways. When we struggle to do this, it's a sign of illness or dysfunction.

This doesn't mean we're broken or beyond repair; it simply means we're responding naturally to our circumstances and need to give ourselves time, space, and compassion. We can examine what we need to help us move through challenges, let go, and find a semblance of order in the chaos.

You might be surprised by the variability in your capacity, or you might already be aware of it. There are times when you'll accomplish a lot with few mistakes, and other times when it feels like you're stuck, spinning your wheels without making progress. This ebb and flow is a regular part of being human in the 21st century.

In writing this book, my mission is to remind you that we are all co-creating our future, at least to some degree. More specifically, I hope to convince you that you can play a more conscious role in creating your own future, and in becoming a healthier and happier, fully actualized human being. I hope you can see that this is also the best thing you can do for the earth and humanity 'at large'.

Ultimately, there is always only "now," and there has never been a better time to act than "right now." The choices we make--how and where we focus our attention--matter. The energy you bring to life impacts your individual experience and the broader collectiveness of humanity.

Where Can We Go from Here?

The future is always uncertain. The robots are coming. The sky is still falling...

...Actually, in the time it took me to write this book, the robots have arrived.

With so many new technologies on the horizon and so many factors contributing to the complexity of our world, it's easy to lose focus. It's natural to feel overwhelmed by the questions, the uncertainty, and the constant demands on our attention. Our systems are being driven to a state of overload more and more each day. If you don't take deliberate action to manage this, you risk being swept away or remaining stuck, like a rat in a cage, for years or even a lifetime.

I invite you; I give you permission, and I "double-dog dare" you to take action today. Then take action again tomorrow. Join our free support community or find another group of growth-minded peers.

Visit your local library, dog park, or choir. Take up yoga, try neurographic art, explore HeartMath, or learn to snowboard. Do something to disrupt your current pattern and build momentum toward shifting your life.

Start small or start big. Just set a goal based on your best and most informed 'guess' and start. Track your progress and reflect. Adjust and begin again.

Celebrate and document your successes. Tell people or at least one person about your experiences and your feelings about your experiences. I want to hear about them, so if you don't have someone else to share them with, please share them with me.

Send an email, post on social media, or tell a friend. It's a big deal to be alive! It's a big deal to be able to self-reflect and steer the wheel of your own ship.

Don't let life pass you by without deciding what you want and at least trying to achieve it. You are capable of so much more than you think.

Remember to reflect on how far you've come along the way.

Look how far you have come!

Give yourself a mental high-five and a pat on the back for caring enough about your future and destiny to make this journey with me. Taking responsibility for your life is no small feat! Many people never dare to consciously take the wheel and steer their own life.

Pause, take a deep breath, and anchor this feeling in your body right now. You are making progress! You are taking steps to improve your life, and in doing so, you are choosing a better future for all of humanity and consciousness. This is no small thing!

The Shift. Own your emotions; Own your life.

Keep Laughing!

Life is much too important to take it too seriously.

No one gets out of this life alive. Death is the great equalizer that comes to us all eventually. So, live your life with vim and vigor, but don't get addicted to drama. Don't let it suck you into the deep recesses of suffering and decay before it's your time. Make it a habit to let go of stress regularly, or it will get the best of you, especially in our modern age.

One of the tools that has helped me through some of the darkest times has been stand-up comedy. I think stand-up comedians are some of the most underappreciated teachers and healers in human societies and our ability to find humor in tragedy and be amused by the absurdities of life is one of the things that makes us resilient and also lovely to be around.

Laughing yoga teaches we can use laughter to shift our neurochemistry even if we are not perceiving anything funny or humorous. Studies show that even fake laughter can have a positive impact on our chemical state and help us become calmer and more coherent. Fake laughter, especially in a group, often leads to genuine laughter. In either case it is a great way to practice deeper breathing, relaxing, and getting more comfortable with silliness. Regular laughter is a delightful way to cultivate vagal tone and improve your emotional fitness.

The Shift. Own your emotions; Own your life.

Take Those Next Steps...

Remember, you are wiser than you think. Your body carries the programming of thousands of years of survival. Many have endured what you're going through in their own ways, and some have risen from their struggles to achieve incredible things. This is your life--embrace it fully.

Now that we've reached the end of this journey together, you're ready to begin. I have an online community where we'd love to welcome you. We're building a global network of like-minded individuals who are committed to empowerment and wellness, rather than disease and dysfunction. Come join us--we need you. And whatever you decide to do, remember: You've got this.

You are worthy of your own love. Give yourself a little bit more.

This is The Beginning...

Keep the Momentum Going!

We've done a lot of good work together--planted seeds of change, built a foundation for self-mastery, and set some big things in motion. But here's the deal: the journey doesn't stop here. In fact, this is where it really begins. Staying on track means continuing to engage with the work we've started, connecting with others on the same path, and making sure that what you've learned really sticks.

Repetition works. Iterations are the secret to progress. The more you follow up, engage with a like-minded community, and review what you've learned, the more likely you are to see real, lasting transformation. Repeat what is working and change what is not working.

Form or Join a Community: There IS Strength in Numbers

Going alone can be tough. That's why forming or joining a like-minded community can make all the difference in sticking with your personal growth journey. Research shows that when we're part of a supportive community, we're more likely to stay committed to our goals, especially when things get tough.

When you surround yourself with people who are also striving for growth, you create a network of accountability and support that keeps you on track. Whether it's joining an online group, participating in forums, or even forming your own local meetup, being in community amplifies your efforts. Plus, let's be honest--doing the work together is usually just more fun. You get to share the wins, support each other through challenges, and keep the momentum going.

Review what you've learned!

Now, let's talk about repetition again. You've probably heard that old saying, "Repetition is the mother of all learning," and it turns out, science totally agrees. Studies on spaced repetition--the idea that reviewing information at intervals helps with long-term retention--show that we're more likely to remember and apply what we've learned when we go over it more than once. I like to think of repetitions more as iterations and try to make slight adjustments along the way whenever I see where there is room for improvement.

The Shift. Own your emotions; Own your life.

If you really want the ideas and tools we've covered to take root and flourish, you will need to keep coming back to them.

Review your notes, revisit key takeaways, and re-engage with the content--whether it's through re-reading chapters, listening to podcasts, or discussing with others in the community. Find new variations and try slightly different ways to see what works best for you all along the way. The more you engage with the material, the more it becomes a part of you, rather than just something you read once and forgot.

Follow-Up and Stay Engaged.

We've all been there: finishing a great book or course, feeling pumped up, and then… "crickets". Life happens, and it's easy to fall back into old routines. But here's the thing--following up is essential to keeping the momentum alive.

This is where I come in! Stay connected, keep engaging with the community, and follow up regularly--whether it's through online discussions, Q&As, or joining live events. This not only helps you retain what you've learned, but it also makes the process of growth more interactive and dynamic. Plus, we're all here to support each other--no one's doing this alone.

The bottom line? The work doesn't stop here. The best way to keep moving forward is by staying engaged, reviewing what you've learned, and connecting with a community that shares your values. So don't let this be the last step--let it be the first of many. Join the conversation, stay connected, and let's keep the momentum going together.

Time flies like an arrow; fruit flies like a banana.

The Shift. Own your emotions; Own your life.

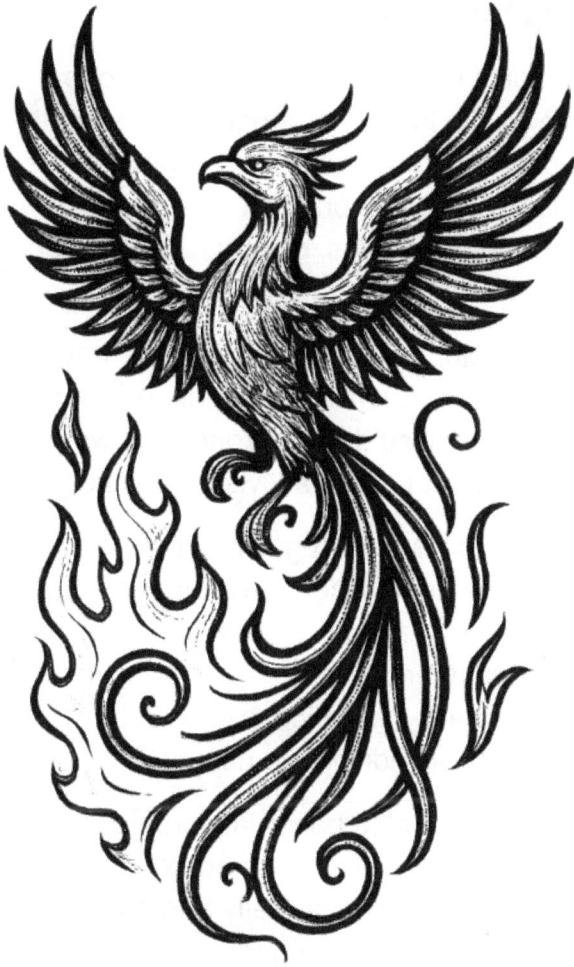

More Real People Who Inspire Me:

Maya Angelou: The Poetic Phoenix

Maya Angelou's life story is another great one of transforming pain, loss, and struggle into something powerful, beautiful, and transcendent. Her journey wasn't easy, but like the golden phoenix, she continually rose from the ashes of her hardships, recreating herself and using her voice to uplift others.

As a child, Angelou endured unspeakable trauma, leaving her silent for years. But from that silence, she found her voice, a voice that would echo around the world, inspiring millions through her poetry, activism, and storytelling.

At the age of eight, Maya Angelou was sexually abused by her mother's boyfriend. After revealing the abuse to her family, her abuser was killed, leading to an overwhelming sense of guilt and fear. As a result, Angelou became mute for nearly five years. Her voice, a key part of her identity, was lost, and she withdrew into herself.

Even in silence, Angelou began absorbing the world around her in a new way. She immersed herself in books, learning to communicate internally and mentally preparing for her eventual rebirth. During this period, her inner world grew stronger, and though the pain silenced her, it also laid the foundation for the remarkable writer and storyteller she would later become.

After years of silence, Angelou found her voice again through the encouragement of a teacher and a family friend, Mrs. Bertha Flowers, who introduced her to literature and poetry. It wasn't just a return to speaking; it was the

The Shift. Own your emotions; Own your life.

beginning of Maya Angelou's journey into becoming a poet, a storyteller, and eventually one of the most influential voices in American literature.

Even in her later years, Maya Angelou continued to evolve, remaining a powerful voice for justice, equality, and self-love. She took on roles as a mentor, teacher, and elder stateswoman of poetry, inspiring new generations to push back against societal limitations and to rise from their own challenges.

Amanda Gorman: The Poet of Progress

Amanda Gorman, the youngest inaugural poet in U.S. history, also demonstrates the transformative power of resilience, creativity, and self-expression. Her journey began with a speech impediment that made speaking--let alone public performance--a daunting challenge. As a child, Amanda faced moments of self-doubt, grappling with feelings of inadequacy. Yet rather than letting her challenges define her, she embraced them as opportunities to grow and develop her voice.

Through years of dedication, Amanda honed her craft as a poet and orator, using mindfulness, practice, and emotional regulation to navigate the anxiety that often accompanies public speaking. She found solace and strength in the written word, turning vulnerability into her superpower. For Amanda, poetry became not just an art form but a tool for transformation--a way to channel emotions, process experiences, and inspire others.

The Shift. Own your emotions; Own your life.

Amanda's story is one of self-mastery through creativity and discipline. By transforming her fears into fuel for growth, she has shown that challenges can be the foundation for greatness. Her life story reminds us that emotional resilience and purpose-driven action are cultivated through small, consistent efforts. Amanda inspires us to embrace our unique stories, knowing that even the smallest voices can spark monumental change.

Gabrielle Reece: Grace and Strength in Motion

Gabrielle Reece's life story is also a testament to resilience and the pursuit of excellence. As a professional volleyball player, she reached the pinnacle of her sport, becoming a symbol of strength and grace. Her journey wasn't without challenges. Gabrielle faced injuries that threatened her career, moments of doubt about her path, and the immense pressure of living in the public eye. Through it all, she turned to tools like mindfulness, breathwork, and journaling to process her emotions and maintain focus. She also embraced physical movement not just as a profession, but as a way to regulate her mental state and stay connected to her goals.

Off the court, Gabrielle has built a career as a fitness advocate, author, and speaker. Her ability to balance multiple roles--athlete, wife, mother, and mentor-- demonstrates her skill in goal stacking: aligning her personal and professional ambitions to create a fulfilling and impactful life. She has inspired countless people to take ownership of their health and find empowerment through discipline and self-care.

Laird Hamilton: Riding the Biggest Waves

Laird Hamilton, a legendary big-wave surfer, is known for his fearless approach to conquering some of the most dangerous waves on the planet. But his path to success has been anything but smooth. Growing up in Hawaii, Laird faced a difficult childhood, marked by feelings of being an outsider and the struggles of navigating a turbulent family life. These experiences shaped his drive to prove himself and find solace in the ocean.

Laird's relentless pursuit of excellence has been fueled by a combination of physical conditioning, mental toughness, and innovative thinking. He has developed groundbreaking techniques and equipment, like the hydrofoil surfboard, that have revolutionized the sport. To manage the emotional highs and lows of such a risky career, Laird relies on tools like controlled breathing, visualization, and cold exposure-- practices that help him stay calm under pressure and recover from the physical and emotional toll of his pursuits.

Gabrielle and Laird: The Power of Partnership

Together, Gabrielle Reece and Laird Hamilton embody the concept of polarity: the balance of contrasting energies that creates something greater than the sum of its parts.

The Shift. Own your emotions; Own your life.

Gabrielle's structured, disciplined approach complements Laird's adventurous and intuitive mindset, allowing them to support and challenge each other in unique ways. Their shared commitment to health and personal growth has not only strengthened their relationship but also inspired their joint ventures, including fitness programs and wellness retreats that help others unlock their potential.

As a couple, they demonstrate how shared goals and mutual respect can amplify individual strengths. Their ability to navigate challenges together--whether it's balancing demanding careers or raising a family--highlights the importance of communication, adaptability, and a deep understanding of each other's needs.

Jacqueline Novogratz: Dignity in Action

Jacqueline Novogratz's story is one of transformation and impact. Her journey began with a defining moment: spotting her old blue sweater being worn by a young boy in Rwanda. This encounter sparked a realization about the interconnectedness of the world and the unintended consequences of well-meaning actions. Determined to make a difference, Jacqueline founded Acumen, a nonprofit organization that uses patient capital to address global poverty.

Building Acumen wasn't easy. Jacqueline faced skepticism, failures, and the emotional toll of witnessing extreme poverty. Yet, she persevered, drawing strength from tools like storytelling, deep listening, and a commitment to continuous learning. By embracing failure as feedback, she

The Shift. Own your emotions; Own your life.

has created a model that empowers communities to solve their own problems with dignity and accountability.

Chris Anderson: Spreading Ideas Worth Sharing

Chris Anderson, best known for his leadership of TED, has transformed the platform into a global phenomenon that amplifies "ideas worth spreading." His journey, however, was marked by early struggles, including financial setbacks and the challenge of maintaining his vision in the face of uncertainty. Chris's ability to stay focused on long-term goals, paired with his talent for creating environments where others can shine, has been key to his success.

Chris's emotional resilience is rooted in tools like reflection, strategic thinking, and fostering meaningful connections. By prioritizing clarity and purpose, he has built a legacy that inspires millions of people worldwide to think bigger and act with intention.

Jacqueline and Chris: A Shared Mission

Together, Jacqueline Novogratz and Chris Anderson exemplify the power of aligned goals and shared values. Their partnership is a testament to the impact of mutual support and a common vision. While they each pursue distinct missions, their ability to hold space for each other's growth and celebrate each other's successes has amplified their individual and collective impact.

Their relationship highlights the importance of balancing personal ambition with partnership, showing that true success often comes from lifting each other up. By combining their strengths and staying true to their values, they've created a legacy that inspires change and innovation on a global scale.

The Shift. Own your emotions; Own your life.

➤

INVITATION TO ACTION:

Break Your Inertia: Identify one area in your life where you feel stuck--whether it's a goal, habit, or project. Commit to taking one small action in the next 24 hours. Remember, it's the first step that breaks the inertia. Even the smallest movement will create momentum.

Reduce Your Resistance: List the internal and external obstacles that create resistance in your progress. Consider which of these are mental blocks (like fear or self-doubt) and which are physical (like time or resources). For each, come up with a small, actionable solution to reduce resistance.

Check Your Alignment: Review your top three current goals. Are they aligned with your values and long-term purpose? Next to each goal, write the core value it represents. If any goals feel misaligned, take time to realign or replace them with ones that better reflect who you are.

The Shift. Own your emotions; Own your life.

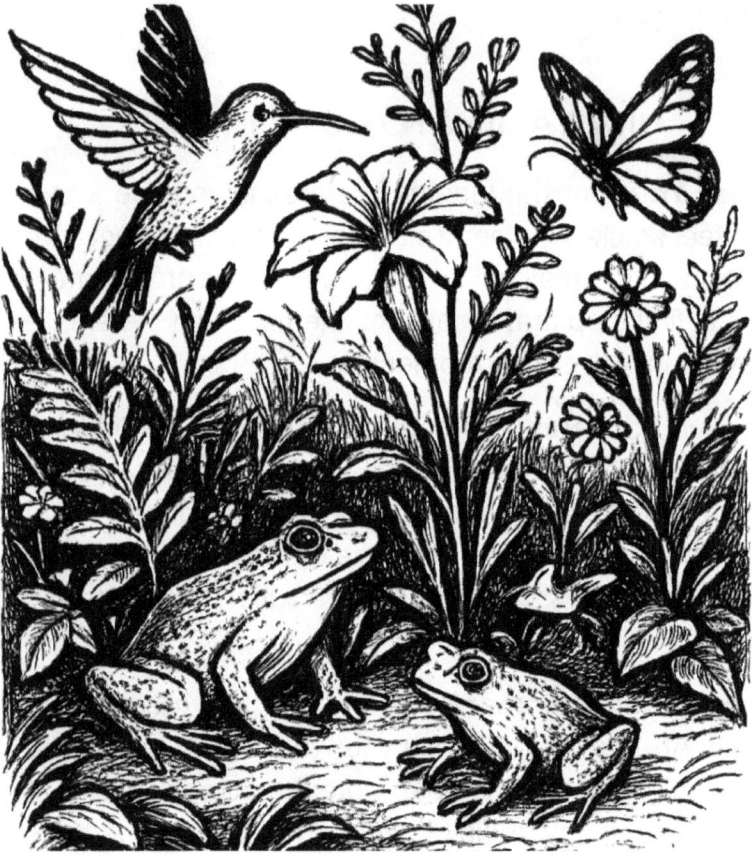

The Tale of the Unlikely Garden

In a quiet village, nestled between rolling hills, there lived a young woman named Marla. Marla was known for her perfectly kept garden.

Every flower was planted in straight rows. Every bush was always trimmed to perfection, and every tree grew exactly as she intended. Her garden was her pride and joy, a place

The Shift. Own your emotions; Own your life.

where she could control every detail and predict every outcome.

One spring, a wild and unexpected storm swept through the village. The winds howled, and the rain poured with such fury that it seemed as if the heavens were determined to wash everything away.

Marla watched helplessly from her window as the storm tore through her beloved garden, uprooting flowers, bending trees, and leaving chaos in its wake.

When the storm finally passed, Marla stepped out into the garden. Her heart was heavy with despair. The once perfect rows were now a tangled mess, and her carefully tended plants lay scattered and broken.

She spent days mourning the loss, unable to face the destruction that had befallen her sanctuary.

But as the days turned into weeks, something remarkable began to happen. Amid the ruins, Marla noticed new life starting to emerge. Wildflowers she had never planted began to sprout in unexpected places. A vine, carried by the storm from a distant hill, took root in the corner of her garden, wrapping itself around the damaged trees and bringing them back to life. The chaotic tangle of plants began to grow into a vibrant, colorful landscape that Marla had never imagined.

At first, Marla resisted the natural beauty of this new garden. It was nothing like the orderly rows she had carefully planned. But as time went on, she began to grow an appreciation for the beauty in the wildness.

The garden had a life of its own now, one that was unpredictable and full of surprises. The wildflowers brought

The Shift. Own your emotions; Own your life.

bees and butterflies, the vines provided shelter for birds, and the once rigid garden had transformed into a living, breathing ecosystem.

Marla realized that the storm had given her a gift--a garden that was far more beautiful and alive than anything she could have created on her own. The storm had taught her that life doesn't always go according to plan, and that sometimes, the most beautiful things come from the unexpected.

From that day on, Marla tended her garden with a new sense of wonder. She stopped trying to control every detail. Instead, Marla let the garden grow as it wished, guiding it gently but leaving room for the wildness that had transformed it. In letting go of her need to control the garden, and just allowing it to grow on its own, Marla found a peace she had never known.

The End.

About the Author:

Let's go all the way back to the beginning. I was born in Washington state and spent the first handful of years of my life picking berries, hunting for tadpoles and frogs, making fudge for fairies, learning to eat crab…it was a good childhood. My mother and I were poor, but she kept me fed and let me do whatever I wanted. I was reading well by age four.

I had quite a few near-death experiences by the time I was five. Left alone my first night home. Nearly drown in bucket of water the next day. Left in the car…Playing on train tracks and in tunnels at age three. Climbing dangerously high up more than one tree…most of these I only remember vaguely, if at all.

I was diagnosed with incurable, chronic systemic autoimmune disease before puberty and told I would not live to 50, and that my life would probably involve a lot of extra pain and suffering. Right now, I am 54 and though I do live with chronic pain and my fair share of suffering, I do not believe our current health care system is on the right track when it comes to chronic and systemic disease.

Today, having an autoimmune disease is so commonplace that no one 'bats an eye' at it, but it was almost unheard of in the early 1980s. I was also very shy and had a hard time relating to people my age.

For nearly twelve years, from puberty until just before I became a mother, I struggled with a painful, disfiguring rash (chronic urticaria, or hives) that frequently covered much of my body, including my face. I also developed rheumatoid arthritis, psoriasis, digestive issues, negative thought patterns, sclerosis, neuralgia, and several other conditions. I started drinking alcohol and smoking tobacco at age 12, along with other self-harming behaviors.

Many of these issues persist today, but I have come to recognize that they are largely the result of dissociating from my true nature, suppressing and repressing my emotions, and not feeling safe enough to become fully self-actualized.

Now, as many as 80%-90% of Americans suffer from at least one condition that falls under the umbrella of 'autoimmunity.' This term is a catch-all for a systemic dysfunction that is still poorly understood by our medical-industrial complex.

I hope that we will come to a more functional and useful understanding of the wisdom inherent in our body systems and learn to get out of our own way so that we can heal, both individually and collectively.

In fifth grade, I was extensively tested and told I was 'almost a genius' (missed it by two points or something like that). In sixth grade, I was given double or triple the workload of my peers and then skipped ahead a few grades.

I was labeled as 'gifted' and a 'Child in Need of Supervision' after my mother tried to have me arrested when she found out I was sexually active at age 13. Shortly after that I was incarcerated for a short time--a couple of weeks at age 13, and a few days again in my later teens.

The principal of the high school I was moved into was a sexual predator who groomed the 'at-risk youth' in his care. Many people in our small town knew about it, including his wife, who was the principal of the grade school I had attended and later became a politician, but no one seemed to care.

When I was informed that I was unlikely to live to 50 and that I would probably live a life of extra pain, disfigurement, and suffering, I remember thinking that was fine with me. I was confident I would be dead before I got to 18. "Only the good die young" and "better to burn out than fade away" were my mottos. I also lived by the cred "Fuck them before they fuck you" for a short time.

I have been a liar and a thief. I have been a victim, perpetrator, martyr, sex worker, bodyworker, healer, artist, businesswoman, musician, student, drug dealer, teacher, substitute, landscaper, and many other basic and complicated archetypes, all numerous times throughout my life.

Right now I am a musician, a songwriter, a singer, an artist, a builder, a philosopher, a snowboarder, a gardener, a photographer, a homeowner, a businesswoman, an author, a hostess, a guide, a consultant, an entertainer, a teacher, a student, a friend, a lover, a daughter, a mother, a sister, an aunt... and more.

Back then, I had no desire to grow old, become less functional, and frail as so many humans seemed to. I had no desire to get married and raise a family in the traditional way I saw many people living life. I was appalled to discover that females were (and still are) considered the 'weaker' sex when I started school and was exposed to television programming.

To my perception, even physically weak females hold much more power than most males. Although I have always enjoyed doing many things that are considered more masculine--fixing things, building things, digging, working

The Shift. Own your emotions; Own your life.

with cars, and practicing martial arts, which was called being a tomboy back then--I also love being a woman.

I now see how much of my draw toward men was a desperate desire for fatherly attention, which I never received. I still see human sexuality, and the dynamic dance between masculinity and femininity, as a great and largely untapped potential power for humanity, but that is a topic for another book.

Throughout my childhood, I read voraciously and wrote avidly. I spoke and read quite well from an unusually young age. Today it's called hyperlexia. I have had an independent spirit for as long as I can remember.

These days that would probably be attributed to neglect, but to be fair, the standards for neglect and abuse were much different for what is now called 'Gen X.' Back then, it was considered bad parenting not to spank, hit, or whip your children, at least sometimes. The neglect and abuse I experienced did make me strong and independent, like many of my generation.

Still, I was, and am, a relatively unique individual. I am an outlier on most data charts. Two standard deviations to the right usually, and occasionally a standard deviation or two to the left of any 'normalcy' bell curve. This is something I have only become increasingly aware of as I age.

Throughout my life, I have been a freelancer and an entrepreneur. In grade school, it was clear to me that I was not 'like other children' and that it was up to me to build a life that would support me. I was the only one I knew who called my mother by her first name instead of 'mom' or 'mommy',' and ' I was one of only a few children I ever met who did not have a father. I tried to sell fossils on the side of the road at age six and fresh vegetables and homemade pies door-to-door around ages eight to eleven.

My grade-school years were mostly wonderful. I played in ditches and streams and rode horses that 'belonged' to other people. I also 'had' a horse of 'my own' for several years named Sundancer. He was the offspring of a somewhat famous Thoroughbred stallion and a wild mustang mare. My mother and I spent some time together teaching him how to 'be useful.' I indulged in my rich imagination, acted out strange rituals, and found escape in reading and writing.

We had goats and ducks, dogs and cats, and always had a large garden and picked fresh fruit in local orchards to store in the root cellar. I also spent a lot of time trying to care for wounded birds and dogs I found, leaving treats and stones for fairies, building clubhouses, digging kivas and caves, and looking for secret underground structures and pots of gold at the end of rainbows.

By age 15 I was legally emancipated from my mother and working as a waitress--until I discovered the black market and 'outlaw life' that is. Around age 17, I was 'adopted' by a gang of bikers. I spent the next 2-3 years learning a lot about life from a man I still refer to as 'my biker sugar daddy' who was, and still is, for all intents and purposes, the closest thing to a father I had (perhaps until just recently, as I do have some contact with my actual biological father now).

In my late teens and young adult life, amidst some waitressing and other 'regular' jobs (which I lied about my age to get), and many less 'legitimate' jobs, I also did housecleaning, landscaping, and started several small businesses to try to earn a living. Most of them failed by societal standards, but in my 30s, I was able to run my own

The Shift. Own your emotions; Own your life.

Massage Therapy and Bodywork business and became an eBay power-seller for more than a decade.

In my mid-teens, living mostly 'on the streets,' I had discovered the black market, psychedelics, and other substances, and built a well-trusted reputation as someone who could always 'get what you need.' In my mid-20s, I became a licensed massage therapist and bodyworker, and a 'professional student' for 15 years, earning dozens of certificates, a Bachelor's and two Master's degrees. All of this allowed me to raise my son without putting him into regular daycare.

It's fair to say I have seen a lot of the 'soft grimy underbelly' of society. Many people from all walks of life have shared their deepest, and often darkest secrets with me. I have built a fairly customized life that has been overall quite fulfilling on many levels.

Giving birth to my son and becoming a mother changed everything for me, as it does for most parents. I was inspired to live a longer and more positive life and determined to get healthy. I studied many healing modalities and discovered my body has a great capacity to heal. I became interested in cleansing, fasting, breathwork, and moving meditations.

Skip ahead to my late 40's when I experienced a somewhat typical mid-life meltdown. At age 51 I realized I am autistic by today's standards as it felt like my entire life and everything I thought I knew about myself and about humanity shifted during the pandemic.

Now, a couple years after that, I continue to realize I also struggle with ADHD and now, pretty severe complex PTSD. Of course, all of these are labels. The labels are made up and they will change.

The Shift. Own your emotions; Own your life.

These things are wired into my nervous system, and also, they are always changing, just like everything else. I currently identify as 'neurospicy' and enjoy exploring what that means, especially when it comes to managing my emotions and my relationships.

In more recent years, I have come to a better understanding of how neurodivergence has played a role in my family and personal history, and how my autoimmunity and systemic inflammation have also been intertwined with this and my attempts to please my mother. I would be remiss if I didn't mention that my mother is a very pleasant person almost all the time. I am frequently grateful for that and for her presence in my life.

Why I Wrote This Book

Emotional dysregulation has been at the heart of many of my personal challenges, and that has led me down a path of healing and trying to help others learn to heal. I know from decades of experience, many children and adults suffer from a lack of emotional fitness. I know these skills are teachable, and that with practice any of us can improve our lives by improving our ability to feel our emotions without being overwhelmed or ruled by them. Children and adults can learn to use these tools and techniques.

I grew up like many humans, with a mix of positives and negatives. We had a lot of puppies and ducks. Although I was cared for and well-fed, my relationship with my mother was fraught with unhealthy attachments and boundaries, and my father was absent from my life altogether.

The Shift. Own your emotions; Own your life.

My parents were themselves at least in part the products of abuse and neglect, like so many children and parents are, which makes it difficult to fully comprehend their actions in this rapidly changing technological age. Each generation lives in a different time and has its own unique history, but we're all doing the best we can with what we have. My parents were no exception.

I learned early on to override my own feelings and needs to attune to my mother's needs and those of others around me. I spent a lot of my life swinging between victim, savior, and perpetrator mindsets. It wasn't until just a few years ago that I really saw how I was doing this from a new perspective, and realized this wasn't the way to love or be loved. My perspective has since shifted dramatically at several points in my life, as perspectives of life-long learners are prone to do.

My maternal grandfather was a successful engineer, and early on, I noticed the stark differences between how the rich and poor live, think, and act. Even at a young age, it was striking to me. This gave me a unique perspective on how our mindset determines our actions, which ultimately determines the quality of our lives. To be clear, my grandfather was wealthy, but he was also a "functional alcoholic", and not very happy much of the time. This was fairly standard for his generation, I think.

When I was 13, my mother rejected me, and I was briefly incarcerated as a ward of the state. This experience changed me profoundly. Being locked in a steel and cement cage and shunned by those charged with instilling love and healthy relationships has extreme and long-lasting effects. It damages both the humans in the cages and those who hold the keys. One of my deepest passions is to help humanity improve how we handle civil disobedience, sexuality, and the treatment of abandoned, neglected, and abused children.

Most children in juvenile detention centers have been neglected, abused, and often have traumatic brain injuries or other significant issues before they are locked up. This makes their incarceration even more insane and cruel. Most of them are dysregulated at the time if they are committing a crime. Most of them are there, at least in part due to emotional dysregulation of some or all of the adults who are in charge of their care and protection. This is how generational trauma becomes systemic, societal trauma.

Right now, we seem to be in a real mental illness crisis, at least in American culture. Suicide rates have dramatically increased, especially among young men. As a mother and a daughter and a sister, I feel compelled to DO something. This book, and doing the work of shifting myself, is one facet of my progress towards this aim.

My Personal Journey to Healing

I dropped out of high school and lived on the streets for several years during my teens. During that time, I witnessed and experienced things that many in mainstream society remain sheltered from. I was raped, beaten, arrested, ripped off, trusted, and betrayed--more than once. I was eventually taken in by a group of bikers in my late teens, where I learned more about crime and how the black market operates. "Raised by wolves" and "yes, literally in a barn" is how I often describe this aspect of my upbringings. Like everything in life, it had its positives and its negatives.

I became intimately familiar with the part of life that mainstream culture pretends not to see but that is always

The Shift. Own your emotions; Own your life.

present, lurking in the alleys and weaving through every facet of our world. Many of the details of those times are simmering in another book, for another time.

In my twenties I became a mother and began exploring various healing modalities in an effort to keep myself and my son healthy. I started a business selling herbs, oils, and cosmetic supplies, became a massage therapist, and continued my studies in martial arts, moving meditation, dance, and yoga.

My interests expanded to include biochemistry, anatomy and physiology, neuroscience, patterns of earth and humanity, ceramics, site-specific art, and storytelling. I even completed a year and a half of premed study with the intention of becoming a surgeon, but I ultimately left the program when I realized the medical school I was attending was deeply influenced by big pharma and insurance companies.

 Helping people within that system would have forced me to compromise my values, so I chose to walk away.

In my thirties, I earned two master's (MA) degrees--one in Business and Organizational Management and another in Special Education with an emphasis on severe disabilities, savant skills, and autism. I developed a deep interest in biochemistry, neurodivergence, human psychology, and brain science. I became fascinated by the way stories and symbols influence our subconscious, shaping our identities and creating patterns that determine our behaviors and outcomes in life.

Our mindset, the stories we tell ourselves, and the way we interpret the stories others tell us, ultimately shape our beliefs and values. These, in turn, dictate our actions and the kind of life we live.

The Shift. Own your emotions; Own your life.

In every phase of my life, people have shared many stories with me, as I am sure they have with you. When I put all these stories together, I am reminded that most of us struggle with the same sorts of things. Many of these familiar and repeating patterns are the result of the accumulations and stagnations of suppressed and repressed emotions, unprocessed feelings, immature coping strategies, and ineffective tools for self-management.

In my mid-to-late forties, a series of events forced me to confront many of my early traumas from a new perspective. It was more challenging than I had anticipated. I was raped again, publicly shunned, and humiliated for articulating my beliefs which differ from much of mainstream society. I lost my business, most of my friends, and an intimate partnership that had once been new levels of empowering for me but then had become dismal and confusing.

This has been a common pattern in my relationships, and I had already realized this was due to my own trauma-driven responses when I found myself in the same repeating cycle yet again. This rift reopened many past traumas and unhealed wounds, making me more acutely aware of unresolved feelings from my turbulent childhood and the neurodivergent threads that run through my genetic line.

My personal failures and the societal meltdowns around me led to my own systemic meltdown, marked by dysfunctional rage that lasted several years.

I lost my ability to work, and my executive function dwindled to the point where I could barely function a few hours a day. I spent many months wallowing in resentment, blame, and self-pity and weeping uncontrollably. I began preparing for death, halfheartedly and without much logic or plan.

The Shift. Own your emotions; Own your life.

But I am still alive! And so are you! Here we are. We made it this far.

As I go through what I hope will be the final edit of this book, I am in my early-mid 50's and feel as though I could easily thrive for another 40 years or more. Daily yoga, journaling, art therapy, 'belonging walks', sound-healing, singing, and meditation, along with taking full responsibility for my own wellness, are keys for me.

Letting go of resentments, consuming less, cultivating coherence and awareness in my body, asking better questions, eating a diverse range of vegetables and healthy proteins, and caring for my energetic state more proactively have all unlocked new levels of healing in my life.

I have shifted, and I believe you can too. We can all shift.

As Jane Goodall famously pointed out in *The Book of Hope*, it is not a question of 'if' you are making a difference; the question is, what kind of difference are you making? How much of your unique talents and understanding are you cultivating to make a positive difference in this life?

"You cannot get through a single day without having an impact on the world around you. What you do makes a difference, and you have to decide what kind of difference you want to make." —Jane Goodall

References

Below is a curated list of the books, research articles, and authors whose work has helped shape the ideas in this book. Many more could be added, but these were especially influential in crafting The Shift.

Ashford, S. J., & DeRue, D. S. (2018). *Aligning personal and professional goals for coherence and purpose.* Organizational Behavior and Human Decision Processes.

Austin, J., et al. (2014). *The impact of mindfulness meditation, hypnosis, and deep relaxation on the brain's default mode network.* The Neuroscientist.

Barrett, L. F. (2017). *How Emotions Are Made: The Secret Life of the Brain.* Houghton Mifflin Harcourt.

Bishop, G. J. (2019). *Stop Doing That Sh*t: End Self-Sabotage and Demand Your Life Back*.* HarperOne.

Blackie, S. (2022). *Hagitude: Reimagining the Second Half of Life.* September Publishing.

Brown, B. (2021). *Atlas of the Heart: Mapping Meaningful Connection and the Language of Human Experience.* Random House.

Buhr, E. D., et al. (2010). *Circadian rhythms and their effects on physical health, emotional well-being, and cognitive performance.* Nature Reviews Neuroscience.

Burkeman, O. (2012). *The Antidote: Happiness for People Who Can't Stand Positive Thinking.* Faber & Faber.

Clear, J. (2018). *Atomic Habits: An Easy & Proven Way to Build Good Habits & Break Bad Ones.* Avery.

The Shift. Own your emotions; Own your life.

Dana, D. (2018). *The Polyvagal Theory in Therapy: Engaging the Rhythm of Regulation* (S. W. Porges, Foreword). W. W. Norton & Company.

Dana, D., & Porges, S. (2021). *Anchored: How to Befriend Your Nervous System Using Polyvagal Theory*. Sounds True.

Dennis, J. P., & Vander Wal, J. S. (2016). *Cognitive flexibility in managing stress and navigating emotional complexity*. Behaviour Research and Therapy.

Dietrich, A. (2018). *Transient hypofrontality and its role in achieving flow state*. Frontiers in Psychology.

Dweck, C. S., et al. (2019). *Growth-oriented goals and their influence on happiness and emotional resilience*. Personality and Social Psychology Bulletin.

Estés, C. P. (1992). *Warming the Stone Child: Myths and Stories about Abandonment and the Unmothered Child*. Sounds True.

Estés, C. P. (2008). *Joyous Body: Myths and Stories of the Wise Woman Archetype*. Sounds True.

Estés, C. P. (2013). *How to Be an Elder: Myths and Stories of the Wise Woman Archetype*. Sounds True.

Estés, C. P. (2019). *The Gift of Story: A Wise Tale About What Is Enough*. Sounds True.

Ford, B. Q., et al. (2015). *The benefits of acknowledging and accepting emotions over suppression*. Emotion.

Gawdat, M. (2017). *Solve for Happy: Engineer Your Path to Joy*. North Star Way.

Gawdat, M., & Law, A. (2022). *Unstressable: A Practical Guide to Stress-Free Living.* North Star Way.

Gilbert, E. (2015). *Big Magic: Creative Living Beyond Fear.* Riverhead Books.

Gross, J. J., & John, O. P. (2013). *Cognitive reframing and its impact on emotional regulation.* Cognitive Therapy and Research.

Hari, J. (2022). *Stolen Focus: Why You Can't Pay Attention—and How to Think Deeply Again.* Crown.

Hendrix, H., & Hunt, H. L. (2021). *Doing Imago Relationship Therapy in the Space-Between: A Clinician's Guide.* W. W. Norton & Company.

Hollis, J. (2005). *A Life of Meaning: Exploring Our Deepest Questions and Motivations.* Gotham Books.

Hu, J., Zhang, J., Hu, L., Yu, H., & Xu, J. (2021). *Art therapy: A complementary treatment for mental disorders.* Frontiers in Psychology, 12, 686005. https://doi.org/10.3389/fpsyg.2021.686005

Kashdan, T. B., & Rottenberg, J. (2016). *Embracing impermanence for emotional resilience.* The Journal of Positive Psychology.

Katie, B., & Mitchell, S. (2007). *A Thousand Names for Joy: Living in Harmony with the Way Things Are.* Harmony.

Koestner, R., et al. (2017). *The role of intrinsic values in goal setting and life satisfaction.* Motivation and Emotion.

The Shift. Own your emotions; Own your life.

Kotler, S. (2017). *Stealing Fire: How Silicon Valley, the Navy SEALs, and Maverick Scientists Are Revolutionizing the Way We Live and Work*. HarperCollins.

Kotler, S. (2021). *The Art of Impossible: A Peak Performance Primer*. Harper Wave.

Levine, P. A., & Frederick, A. (1997). *Waking the Tiger: Healing Trauma*. North Atlantic Books.

Lieberman, M. D., et al. (2007). *The impact of affect labeling on emotional reactivity and self-control*. Psychological Science.

Locke, E. A., & Latham, G. P. (2002). *Goal-setting theory and its role in motivation and performance*. American Psychologist.

Magsamen, S., & Ross, I. (2023). *Your Brain on Art: How the Arts Transform Us*. Random House.

McGilchrist, I. (2009). *The Master and His Emissary: The Divided Brain and the Making of the Western World*. Yale University Press.

Mennin, D. S., et al. (2018). *Emotional dysregulation and generalized anxiety disorder*. Journal of Anxiety Disorders.

Miller, A. (2005). *The Body Never Lies: The Lingering Effects of Hurtful Parenting*. W. W. Norton & Company.

Miller, D., & Friesen, P. (2006). *Discontinuous change and the concept of tipping points*. Organizational Dynamics.

Oakley, D. A., & Halligan, P. W. (2017). *Hypnosis as a tool for emotional resilience and stress management*. Consciousness and Cognition.

The Shift. Own your emotions; Own your life.

Papadopoulos, R. K., et al. (2015). *The psychological impact of archetypal imagery*. Frontiers in Psychology.

Parnell, L. (2013). *A Therapist's Guide to EMDR: Tools and Techniques for Successful Treatment*. W. W. Norton & Company.

Perry, B. D., & Winfrey, O. (2021). *What Happened to You?: Conversations on Trauma, Resilience, and Healing*. Flatiron Books.

Rothschild, B. (2021). *Revolutionizing Trauma Treatment: Stabilization, Safety, & Nervous System Balance*. W. W. Norton & Company.

Runkle, A. (2022). *Re-Regulated: Set Your Life Free from Childhood PTSD and the Trauma-Driven Behaviors That Keep You Stuck*. Independently Published.

Ryan, R. M., & Deci, E. L. (1985). *Self-determination theory and its implications for autonomy and emotional well-being*. Psychological Inquiry.

Sadhguru (Vasudev, J.). (2016). *Inner Engineering: A Yogi's Guide to Joy*. Spiegel & Grau.

Seijts, G. H., et al. (2015). *Feedback in goal setting and its influence on motivation*. Journal of Applied Psychology.

Steger, M. F., et al. (2010). *The role of internal anchors in emotional resilience*. The Journal of Personality and Social Psychology.

Steger, M. F., et al. (2018). *Purpose and its impact on resilience and well-being*. The Journal of Positive Psychology.

The Shift. Own your emotions; Own your life.

Tonegawa, S., et al. (2011). *Neuroplasticity and the cognitive processes behind quantum leaps*. Nature Reviews Neuroscience.

Trent, T. (2021). *The Girl Who Buried Her Dreams in a Can*. Viking Books for Young Readers.

Urbaniak, K. (2021). *Unbound: A Woman's Guide to Power*. TarcherPerigee.

van der Kolk, B. (2014). *The Body Keeps the Score: Brain, Mind, and Body in the Healing of Trauma*. Penguin Books.

Walker, P. (2013). *Complex PTSD: From Surviving to Thriving*. Azure Coyote Publishing.

Wiest, B. (2020). *The Mountain Is You: Transforming Self-Sabotage into Self-Mastery*. Thought Catalog Books.

The Courageous Hummingbird

One day, deep in the heart of the forest, a great fire began to spread. The flames raged and crackled, threatening to consume everything in their path. All the animals, large and small, watched helplessly as the blaze grew stronger. Some ran in a panic. Others stood frozen with fear. Many simply accepted that nothing could be done to stop the devastation.

Amidst the chaos, a tiny hummingbird darted toward the river. She dipped her beak into the water, carrying just a single drop, and flew back toward the flames. She released her drop of water onto the fire.

Though it seemed insignificant, she didn't stop. Over and over, the hummingbird flew back and forth, tirelessly picking up drops of water and delivering them to the blaze.

The other animals watched her in disbelief. "What are you doing?" asked the elephant. "You're so small, and the fire is so large. You can't possibly make a difference!"

The hummingbird paused only for a moment, hovering in the air as she looked at her fellow creatures. "I'm doing the best I can," she said. And with that, she returned to the river for another drop.

At first, the animals simply stared, but the hummingbird's determination began to stir something within them.

One by one, they started to follow her lead. The elephant used his trunk to suck up water and spray it onto the flames, the deer kicked dirt over the fire, and the birds in the trees flapped their wings to fan the embers away.

The Shift. Own your emotions; Own your life.

Soon, the entire forest was working together, and little by little, the fire's intensity began to wane.

What had seemed like an unstoppable force was now being tamed, all because a tiny hummingbird had the courage to take action.

She didn't wait for others to join her or for someone bigger to solve the problem. She simply did what she could, and her bravery inspired the others to do the same.

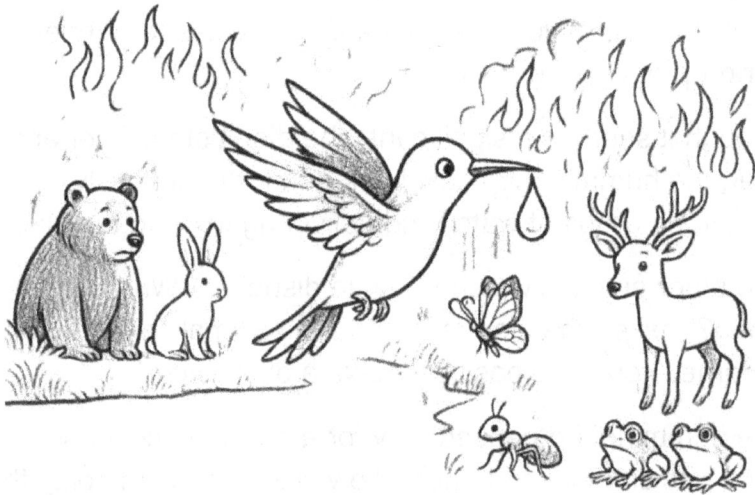

And so we continue to begin again...

www.ingramcontent.com/pod-product-compliance
Lightning Source LLC
Chambersburg PA
CBHW070327090426
42733CB00012B/2386